# Clinical Supervision and
# Mentorship in Nursing

# Clinical Supervision and Mentorship in Nursing

*Edited by*

**TONY BUTTERWORTH**

*and*

**JEAN FAUGIER**

*University of Manchester, UK*

**CHAPMAN & HALL**

London · Glasgow · New York · Tokyo · Melbourne · Madras

Published by Chapman & Hall, 2-6 Boundary Row, London SE1 8HN

Chapman & Hall, 2-6 Boundary Row, London SE1 8HN, UK

Blackie Academic & Professional, Wester Cleddens Road, Bishopbriggs, Glasgow G64 2NZ, UK

Chapman & Hall, 29 West 35th Street, New York NY10001, USA

Chapman & Hall Japan, Thomson Publishing Japan, Hirakawacho Nemoto Building, 6F, 1-7-11 Hirakawa-cho, Chiyoda-ku, Tokyo 102, Japan

Chapman & Hall Australia, Thomas Nelson Australia, 102 Dodds Street, South Melbourne, Victoria 3205, Australia

Chapman & Hall India, R. Seshadri, 32 Second Main Road, CIT East, Madras 600 035, India

Distributed in the USA and Canada by Singular Publishing Group Inc., 4284 41st Street, San Diego, California 92105

First edition 1992
Reprinted 1993

© 1992 Chapman & Hall

Typeset in 10/12pt Times by Columns Design & Production Services Ltd.
Printed in Great Britain by TJ Press (Padstow) Ltd, Padstow, Cornwall

ISBN  0 412 34910 8        1 56593 015 0(USA)

A catalogue record for this book is available from the British Library
Library of Congress Cataloging-in-Publication Data available

# Contents

# Contributors

*Marion Balcombe*   Director, Primary Health Care Education, English National Board for Nursing Midwifery & Health Visiting.

*Phil Barker*   Behavioural Nurse Psychotherapist, Royal Dundee Liff Hospital, Dundee.

*Katie Booth*   Research Fellow, Psychological Medicine Group, University of Manchester, UK.

*Peggy Cooke*   Senior Lecturer, Department of Health Care Studies, Manchester Polytechnic, UK.

*Penny Curtis*   Lecturer, Sheffield Polytechnic, UK.

*Barbara Elliott*   Clinical Nurse Specialist (Research), Booth Hall Children's Hospital, Manchester, UK.

*Jane Merchant*   Executive Director of Nursing and Quality, Manchester Central Hospitals and Community Care N.H.S. Trust, UK.

*Robert Nettleton*   Health Visitor, Stockport Health Authority, UK.

*Brian Pateman*   Teaching Fellow, University of Manchester and District Nurse, Stockport Health Authority, UK.

| | |
|---|---|
| *Sheila Twinn* | Lecturer in Nursing, King's College, University of London, UK. |
| *Peter Wilkin* | Community Psychiatric Nurse, Rochdale Health Authority, UK. |
| *David Woods* | Project Manager – Organizational Design, Liverpool Family Health Services Authority, UK. |
| *Steve Wright* | Consultant Nurse, Nursing Development Unit (Care of the Elderly) Tameside and Glossop Health Authority, UK. |

# PART ONE

# Theoretical Perspectives

## INTRODUCTION

The first section of this book sets the scene for 'supervision' and 'mentorship' in nursing.

It is important to note at the outset that these terms are not the property or province of one particular specialty in nursing but are the proper concern of both clinicians and educators throughout nursing, midwifery and health visiting. It can be argued that various parts of the profession have developed fairly well formed ideas about clinical supervision and mentorship but this does not mean that it 'belongs' to one specialty more than another. Indeed, if a more all embracing view is taken then the various contributions from nursing, midwifery and health visiting to the whole idea of clinical supervision and mentorship are there to be seen.

Midwives have long had 'superintendent midwives'; health visitors and community nurses have prepared their students using fieldwork supervisors and periods of supervised practice for many years. More recently, psychiatric nurses have developed skills in the therapeutic use of self and groupwork; general nurses have developed individualized care through primary nursing, sick children's nurses recognize and work with parents and families as partners, mental handicap nurses have been working within multidisciplinary teams and sharing in common supervision with their non-nurse colleagues. So it is that each of our specialties can show some track record in the subject area.

The authors in this book would suggest that these are all contributory parts to models of mentorship and clinical supervision and in the first part of the book the intention is to show that all those ideas listed above go to form a basis for mentorship and clinical supervision.

In the first chapter Tony Butterworth explores ways in which nursing has started to develop ideas about mentorship and clinical supervision and demonstrates that these ideas are beginning to find expression in the literature. Some 'ground rules' are presented as a beginning and as a basis for action, these are put forward to be criticized and developed further.

In the second chapter Jean Faugier explores a framework on which to base a supervisory relationship and uses a guide within a 'growth and support' model. Supervision in psychotherapy and social work is used to develop some of the elements of the supervisory relationship. The third chapter is concerned with the therapeutic use of self, and its importance in nursing. David Woods discusses the problems of nurses being given sufficient opportunity to work creatively and the need for an appropriate environment in which it might be conducted.

Finally, Katie Booth reviews the literature associated with support and stress reduction. This chapter provides a necessary review of the literature as there is much speculation about the reactive nature of working in nursing, and the repercussion of work upon individual nurses. She highlights the provision of support which has been given to prevent high staff turnover, prevent burnout and increase job satisfaction.

# CHAPTER ONE

# Clinical supervision as an emerging idea in nursing

## Tony Butterworth

Like Leporello, learned men keep a list, but the point is what they lack; while Don Juan seduces and enjoys himself, Leporello notes down the time, the place, and a description. (Kierkegaard)

Writing a book about a constituent part of nursing which is perhaps enjoyed and experienced but not well documented might tempt us, like Leporello, into protracted description without enjoying the pleasures and pain of experience. Hopefully both these things are offered here. It is the intention of this book to demonstrate that exemplars and models of clinical supervision can now be described in nursing which provide both a means of obtaining clinical excellence and an enhancement of the experience of interpersonal relationships. The contributors to this book use the term 'clinical supervision' to embrace a range of strategies in nursing which include preceptorship, mentorship, supervision of qualified practice, peer review and the maintenance of identified professional standards, which gives some indication as to the breadth of subject definition.

There is an emerging literature on the subject of clinical supervision and it is useful to initially consider those influences which have led nursing in this particular direction.

In an attempt to gain independence and achieve mature self-determination, nursing has, with varying degrees of success, attempted to pull away from its origins which tie it amongst other things to the medical profession.

The nursing profession has moved a long way from seeing itself as a less well prepared or educated assistant to the doctor and has become increasingly aware that many roles within nursing and medicine mirror gender roles within society. Nursing could be said to contain a high proportion of expressive roles which carry little attendant power and responsibility. The cost of this lack of professional power is of course reflected in comparatively low financial reward. However, the consequences of being professionally less powerful and in seldom carrying overall responsibility for patient care are manifested in low levels of risk taking and accountability by nurses. Medicine, on the other hand, carries high material rewards and requires the exercise of power and responsibility, which is a common characteristic of male-dominated professions. Interestingly however, whilst doctors cannot avoid overall responsibility, it is possible for them to diffuse the emotional cost of their role through the demands and consequences of working as 'scientists' and by delegation to nursing.

Nursing carries very high emotional cost consequences which are sometimes difficult if not impossible to handle. Menzies (1960) describes very vividly the effects of this emotional cost in relation to the organization of nursing as a social system striving to avoid inherent anxiety by the avoidance of the individual patient or colleague. It is a growing consciousness of issues posed in the change from task-orientated nursing practice which has focused attention on the need for 'support', for the clinical nurse faced with dealing not simply with the patient's psychology, but also her own.

Attempts to de-medicalize nursing are to be found in the literature and are often posited as evidence of a new-found independence (Pearson, 1988; Wright, 1986). As these old ties are cut it might be argued that there is a danger of nursing being left without a source of theoretical nourishment. Interestingly, it appears that the reverse is true, as new areas of knowledge are described and receive explanation. The traditional underpinning influences of the curriculum base of nurse education have been the biological and medical sciences which carry both the kudos of having some 'scientific respectability' but also the inappropriateness and frustrations of reductionism. These constraints have been partially traded off as nursing has moved towards the social sciences and looked for explanations from sociology, psychology and theories in education. In order to accommodate these changes new ways of organizing and presenting nursing care have been established. Most notable of these has been the introduction of the nursing process. The nursing process is seen as a means of ordering nursing care while at the same time being sufficiently flexible to allow changes in theoretical influences and individualized care. Nurses have been urged to reconsider their work within categories which assess, plan and evaluate their work. The key difference in this approach is that it makes task-centred work a thing of the past, and recommends person-centred work with individualized planning as a means to action. Within the process approach, nurses have been urged to form closer and more meaningful relationships with patients and attend to the social, emotional and psychological require- ments of people under their care. Unfortunately, less energy has been spent in helping nurses understand and work with the consequences of close interpersonal exchanges.

In tandem with the nursing process, theories of nursing have appeared which have produced descriptions and paradigms which might provide a base for nursing. The vehicle which takes these theoretical propositions to the clinical setting is the nursing process and within these theories nurses are again urged to 'form a relationship' with patients. Once again the consequences of doing so receives little or no attention from the theoreticians. It follows that nursing has occasionally confused itself and more often alienated its medical and paramedical colleagues by throwing up new theories and action strategies which lay disputable and sometimes confusing territorial claims to new theories and actions which are themselves ill-defined.

It is important to recognize that the more exposed nurses have become to intimate nurse–patient relationships the weaker and more ill-defined have become their protective devices, devices which are not always enabling and have been so clearly identified by Menzies (1960) and Stockwell (1972). In shaking off the paternalist hand of medicine, the protection it provided has gone with it, and little has been done to replace it from within nursing itself. Although nursing has made great strides towards independence (Butterworth, 1990) the attraction of working in teams led by doctors is still evident, offering a paternalism which is more comforting than an independence which carries attendant responsibilities. Small wonder then that nurses are cognitively dissonant about the unprotected opportunism which beckons and the shielded paternalism which frustrates. It is the first contention of this book that models of clinical supervision can be developed in nursing which will protect and improve upon clinical practice and give nursing the necessary support it needs to mature into greater independence.

There are signs that a process of development has already started. A new vocabulary for nurses has appeared in the United Kingdom and is becoming enshrined in information from statutory bodies. A circular from the English National Board for Nurses, Midwives and Health Visitors (ENB), 'Preparation of Teachers, Practitioners/Teachers, Mentors and Supervisors in the Context of Project 2000', appears to be one of the first to recognize an evolutionary change in the nurse to student if not nurse to patient relationship. It is suggested that 'those involved in teaching, facilitating others learning, supervising and assessing, will need to have particular attributes and develop specific competencies'. However, the means to achieving this are less clearly defined. This paper is something of a milestone as it raises and tries to debate a number of terms for the first time. Because of its particular remit, however, it is limited to the changing role of the educationalist and student and does not take the debate into the more general arena of practice. This is a pity, as qualified and experienced nurses are equally in need of similar consideration and it is a second contention of this book that clinical supervision is a model which must endure throughout professional life, thus providing a supportive as well as an educative purpose. An example of supportive supervision is postulated by Wright (1986) when he argues:

> It seems logical to assume that if nurses are to treat patients as human beings, then they in turn need to be treated in the same way by those who manage and educate them. If nurses, through reorganising their working patterns and permitting partnerships with patients, are to have their traditional props pulled from under them, then they need help to find new ways of coping. Opportunities to share feelings, to express views and raise questions are essential, those in management positions at whatever level can provide the new props by an open, supportive and accepting style.

A framework to allow continuous professional development has been provided by the United Kingdom Central Council (UKCC) in their report on post-registration and practice (1990). Its working group had as one of its terms of reference:

> to devise a coherent and comprehensive framework incorporating the standards and principles of education and practice beyond registration to meet the needs of patients and the health services.

The UKCC presents in its report a model of the continuum of practice and suggests that

> a form of post-registration education must occur at least every three years—practitioners have no end point in their need to maintain and develop standards of practice.

It should therefore be possible to devise a model of continuous supervision throughout professional life and accord with requirements of the professional body.

There is a concomitant debate to be found within the Project 2000 proposals being put forward by the Colleges of Nursing, wherein a number of key words can be identified as they gain a more general acceptability. It is necessary to consider two of these key words in this first chapter, namely, mentorship and clinical supervision.

## MENTORSHIP

The role of mentor has gained a new prominence, particularly within educational programmes being developed within Project 2000. Not surprisingly this is territory already explored by American nurses. Darling (1984), one of the pioneers of mentorship in the United States, has gone so far as to devise a system for measuring mentorship potential (Darling MMP2), and has outlined the characteristics of 'good mentors'. These include being:

- an envisioner: giving the learner a picture of what nursing can be like;
- a standard prodder: pushing the learner to achieve high standards; and
- a challenger: making the learner look more closely at her skills and the decisions she makes.

Other writers also emphasize this active educational element. Puetz (1985) describes mentors as possessing several specific functions, including serving as teachers, sponsors, hosts, exemplars and counsellors. Mentors are seen as sharing their experience, thus teaching the best way of doing things, enhancing their protégés' skills and furthering their intellectual ability. One could be forgiven for thinking that this approach is a long way from those less certain, more facilitative models traditionally employed in psychotherapy and social work. It is not surprising that nursing, a profession which finds itself uncomfortable with uncertainty, is attracted to models arrogant enough to claim that mentors or supervisors know the best way of doing things, and have it within their capabilities to enhance skills and further their intellectual development.

Such complex developments are better considered as a product of growth through interaction in a safe and stimulating relationship based on openness and trust, and are as much the responsibility and achievement of the supervisee as of the supervisor. Models of mentorship in which students are merely the object simply mirror the process of clinical nursing in which things are done to patients without them being active in the partnership. Burnard (1989), advocating the role of mentor to district nurses, describes a paradigm proposed by Darling (1984) in which she identifies three aspects to the role of mentor, inspirer, investor and supporter, and suggests that within the role of mentor it is possible to model effective nursing practice. Such a proposition places this aspect of the role of mentor outside that of traditional nurse educator in the United Kingdom. The nurse educator has often become deskilled through lack of practice contact and cannot therefore act as a model of good practice. This is not to criticize, rather to illustrate an evolution in the way that nurse educators have moved away from the practice setting. There have been a number of alternative suggestions, however, which see a role for a teacher/practitioner who might combine clinical skills with teaching (Jarvis and Gibson, 1985). Darling's second aspect of mentoring, 'Investment', suggests that each learner has worth and a measure of potential that can be encouraged, developed and refined in tandem with a mentor. This bears some comparison to the Rogarian view (Rogers, 1951) that for a relationship to progress there must be warm positive unconditional regard, a proposition well known to those involved in counselling. A Rogarian model has no strong base in nursing although the profession has flirted with it in recent times by encouraging nurses to form 'nurse–patient relationships'. Equally, interpersonal skills have been explored in nursing curricula, although the method of acquiring them has not been without criticism.

The third part of the triangle of mentorship is that of supporter. Burnard (1989) suggests that this requires the skills of active listening and empathy. It could be hypothesized that for a student to be trained in a learning environment which encourages these skills will lead to qualified nurses who will foster similar therapeutic exchanges between nurses and patients.

There remains some work to be done on who might be the most suitable mentor 'material'. Such a demanding role obviously requires a competence over and above that of simply being able to function as a trained nurse. A number of concerned commentators in nursing have pointed out the need to be aware of the tremendous importance of choosing those who act as mentors and supervisors. Burnard (1988) highlights the likelihood that

> the relationship between student and mentor also invokes transference, particularly as the mentor is already cast in the role of 'expert' by the very fact that she is a mentor. All this suggests that mentors should be chosen very carefully. Who should be doing the choosing remains a question for debate.

Some writers are in little doubt as to who are most appropriate to act as suitable supervisors. Pembrey (1980) points out the need to have the most able nurses in terms of clinical supervision at ward level. This of course demands the development of a system which will provide a career structure and suitable stimulation in the clinical situation in order to keep the most able nurses practising.

## CLINICAL SUPERVISION

It is possible to find considerable literature on clinical supervision in professions such as psychology, social work and counselling but there is little of substance in nursing. There are exceptions. Midwifery has a long history of clinical supervision and it is possible to find models in health visiting and district nursing but these are often limited to the education of students and do not necessarily extend into qualified practice. There is little literature on supervision in mainstream general nursing and what there is is related to the maintenance of standards rather than to encouragement and personal growth; in this context the model of the superior/novitiate relationship springs to mind. Indeed it is suggested by Hill (1989) that people at work tend to think of their supervisors as authoritarian and that the whole concept of supervision is linked conceptually to an authority figure. This is a pity, because clinical supervision is much wider and more generous in its intentions.

Peer support is often given as an example of supervision carried out by nurses, and most nurses would agree that this occurs regularly on an informal basis although few have constructed the opportunity to formalize peer support to the level found in nurse development units. An example of informal peer support is the 'tea break/tear break', often used as a way of letting colleagues share in stressful clinical experiences which have affected nurses in their working day. From this, nurses gain sympathy but also feedback on how they dealt with a particular situation.

Supervision is often negatively associated with more traditional disciplinary dealings between managers and their staff. These dealings are seen as punitive and can carry impressions born out of previous negotiations between superiors and novitiates, but this is a narrow definition and more generous interpretations are available. It has been suggested by Platt-Koch (1986) that the goals of supervision are (i) to expand the therapist's knowledge base; (ii) to assist in developing clinical proficiency; and (iii) to develop autonomy and self-esteem as a professional. These suggestions are ones with which the authors of this book would have considerable sympathy, indeed, a third contention of this book is that clinical supervision is an enabling process and involves not penalties but an opportunity for personal and professional growth.

## LESSONS FROM OTHER PROFESSIONS

In her interesting review of the literature on supervision in the caring professions Hill (1989) examines the place of supervision in social work and clinical psychology and expresses surprise that supervision has not gained greater ground in nursing. Westheimer (1977) sees the supervisor in social work as ensuring that scarce human and material resources are used to best advantage for the client, and identifies a role for supervisors in raising social work standards and in the allocation of case work. Hill (1989) makes the point that supervisors in social work appear to act as 'a buffer' between field social workers who provide client service and 'managers/policy makers'. A case could be made that nurses working in a health service with general management structures need a similar provision of buffers. Supervision in clinical psychology and psychotherapy has a long history which touches the roots of these therapeutic schools of thought. Freudians, Rogerians and behaviouralists have all embraced the notion of supervision, with a variety of intensities and purpose. Psychodynamic therapists regard supervision as a fundamental element of their preparation and on-going practice. A condition of qualification and practice for some therapists and counsellors is that students and practitioners alike receive constant and regular supervision. In guidelines issued by the British Association for Counselling those who seek accreditation as counsellors must have undertaken a total of 900 hours of training and practice within which will have been 'two hundred hours of skills development, supervision and case discussion'. In addition prospective applicants will have 'an on-going arrangement for consultation and supervision'.

Clinical psychologists have made some firm statements about the proliferation of those who would call themselves therapists and laid claim to the territory themselves in no uncertain terms. It is not always clear where they gain an authority to act as skill brokers in what has been common territory without ownership. What is clear is that, rather like the process of developing into what is recognizably a competent practitioner, the process of becoming a suitable supervisor is one which does not depend upon, nor is owned by, a particular professional group. In a study by Brammer (1979), in which he looked at teachers, psychotherapists, priests and nurses, it is suggested that factors which allow users to recognize a 'good' person with whom to form an interpersonal relationship do not depend upon a particular school of thought or ideological position. Rather, it is factors related to opportunity for intellectual and personal development which make the difference. These are clearly matters which would have an effect on an individual's potential as a mentor or supervisor.

## SUPERVISION AS A PROTECTIVE DEVICE

It could be argued that supervision may provide a means of protection to nurses. Burnout and work-related stress often feature as a cause for professional concern. The causes of burnout and stress are not yet clear.

Copp (1988) suggests that stress can be viewed as both a stimulus and as a response, and supports Cox's definition (1978) of stress as an imbalance between demand and coping where a stress response results when the individual fails to cope with a stimulus. Freudenburger's definition of burnout (1975) includes 'physical and emotional exhaustion involving the development of negative concepts, negative job attitudes and a loss of concern and feelings for clients'. McCarthy (1985) states:

> Nurses are particularly prone to burn out because of the lack of preparation for coping with emotional stress. They are seldom taught to specify their own needs, and they receive little or no training in interpersonal skills. It is not surprising therefore that many are unable to maintain their initial idealism, caring and commitment and the burn out process ensues.

A variety of proposals have been offered which might make up a means of stress management. These include preventive measures involving relaxation and yoga, and go on to providing more tertiary counselling services for nurses who are experiencing symptoms of burnout. The latter strategy would appear to be less useful, and it may be more important to strengthen nurses in order that they can manage their work more comfortably. As Copp (1988) suggests, 'The ability to reduce stress through individual insight and self awareness may be the best method for nurses to lead more fulfilling lifestyles'. A system of clinical supervision in nursing may be the vehicle for providing this.

### SOME DEFINITION OF TERMS

Having initially suggested that clinical supervision is an umbrella term for many things, it is becoming clear that it is possible to differentiate between clinical supervision, mentorship and role of assessor and preceptor. There is some danger in prescribing tight definitions to terminology when a field of knowledge is in an early period of growth; however, there is some evidence of people wishing to combine the role of mentor and assessor (Northcott, 1989), a view which others might find incompatible. As the terms are therefore receiving some attention by nursing, definitions for the purposes of this book may help to clarify at least four of the terms which will occur repeatedly.

1. Mentor  An experienced professional nurturing and guiding the novitiate.
2. Assessor  An experienced professional making judgements on another's ability to carry out procedures or interactions.

3. Clinical supervision   An exchange between practising professionals to enable the development of professional skills.
4. Preceptor   A teacher or instructor.

## ESTABLISHING GROUND RULES

Having provided the terminology, some positional statement is helpful, if only so that others might knock it down! In a profession which embraces mentorship and supervision it is permissible to identify a number of 'ground rules'.

1. Skills should be constantly re-defined and improved throughout professional life.
2. Critical debate about practice activity is a means to professional development.
3. Clinical supervision offers protection to independent and accountable practice.
4. Introduction to a process of clinical supervision should begin in professional training and education, and continue thereafter as an integral part of professional development.
5. Clinical supervision requires time and energy and is not an incidental event.

These 'ground rules' might be further expanded.

1. Skills should be constantly re-defined and improved throughout professional life.
It is not difficult to accept that once nurses have qualified their skills will continue to develop as more experiences are met and worked through. Current thoughts on post-qualifying professional development in nursing would support this (UKCC, 1990) and it is clear that a learning curve continues for some years after qualification. There must be a point however where new experiences are less common and a plateau in learning is reached. Ten years of clinical experience might well consist of two years of new experiences and personal development followed by eight years in which there are no new challenges needing different solutions. It is possible therefore that there may be stagnation and complacency where no ongoing attention is given to developing skills in qualified staff.

2. Critical debate about practice activity is a means to professional development.
There are limited opportunities for nurses to engage in critical debate about practice activities. Nurses are not expected to set aside time

specifically to consider how best to nurse a patient and his/her family.
Case conferences for nurses are a rare event and yet common enough in
the preparation and education of students. Even within a multidisciplinary setting contributions from nurses are often limited. An example,
although somewhat exaggerated, serves to make the point. In a ward
round medical staff will often agonize over the finer points of diagnosis,
social workers will deliver an analysis of social circumstances, psychologists give a list of mental tests and occupational therapists explicate a
range of rehabilitative programmes. When asked (if asked!) the nurse
might contribute by saying 'slept well' or 'up and about' or 'moved
bowels'. Offerings are limited because nurses are not practised in putting
forward a contribution which will stand up to critical review and grows
from a belief that to be criticized means that your ideas must have been
wrong. This, in turn, is a self-inflicted injury brought about by a process
of education which has not used critical analysis of practice and believes
that there is always a 'right answer'.

Because nurses do not indulge in critical debate as a matter of routine
they are not expected to make a significant contribution to case
conferences. Exposure to case conferences is part of a process of clinical
supervision and can help to develop those skills central to an ability to
participate in critical debate related to practice.

3. Clinical supervision offers protection to independent and accountable
practice.
In recent times a bid for independent and accountable practice has grown
in nursing. This bid has manifested itself in a call for advanced nurse
practitioners and assertions that nurses are responsible and therefore
accountable for their own practice. It is not yet clear if nursing is
professionally equipped to handle the consequences of independence and
responsibility.

Stillwell (1988) has suggested that nurse practitioners need to be sure
that:

1. a nurse can practise safely when patients have open access to their
   extended skills;
2. that an extended/expanded role is acceptable to patients;
3. that an extended/expanded role is acceptable to colleagues.

Advanced practice depends upon proper preparation through education
and skill development. The advanced nurse will need a safe professional
framework in which to practise—what has been called 'protected
autonomy'. This can only be achieved by introducing the concept of
clinical supervision into the profession as a whole, not just to enable the
development of the nurse practitioner role but beginning at first level

nurse training and continuing through to the nurse consultant. The rise of a litigation-minded public and less than total defence of assumed vicarious liability by employers brings an added complication to developing the role of the nurse practitioner. Responsibility for action and more importantly extended action must become part and parcel of nursing's 'professional baggage'. Nurses have a strong professional voice through the Royal College of Nursing and they have made their position clear. Two of their documents, 'Boundaries of nursing' (1988a) and 'Specialties in nursing' (1988b), make the case. The first of these two publications suggests that

> The boundaries of nursing must be able to respond to people's needs. Educational curricula and official guidelines however tend to change relatively slowly. It is nurses themselves who are faced with making the decisions as to what they will, and will not, do, since each nurse is accountable for his or her professional practice.

Clearly there is room for professional growth within these boundaries. The second, 'Specialties in Nursing', makes the case with greater force:

> If the profession of nursing is to reach its ultimate goal of providing relevant nursing care to meet individual patients' needs, then ultimately the role of the nurse specialist is central to its achievement.

This claim builds on propositions earlier in the document that nurse specialists are

> experts in a particular aspect of nursing care—they demonstrate refined clinical practice, either as a result of significant experience or advanced expertise, or knowledge in a branch or specialty.

These are obvious requirements for advanced practice and the profession has laid a claim which determines two steps leading to its realization: expert knowledge or clinical skill, and permission to break the boundaries of previously defined roles. This popular rise in professional development is being matched by policy developments in nurse prescribing (Department of Health, 1989) and new opportunities in post-qualifying education which will lead to advanced practice and new responsibilities.

4.    Introduction to a process of clinical supervision should begin in professional training and education, and continue thereafter as an integral part of professional development.

At the introduction of the Nurses, Midwives and Health Visitors Act in 1979 some debate was raised about the requirement for the maintenance of a 'live' register. In order to stay on the UKCC register, qualified nurses and health visitors have to pay a periodic re-registration fee; however with the exception of midwives no requirement to demonstrate competence is required in order to stay on the register. It has now been argued that some mandatory in-service education should be provided in order that those on the register are aware of research and changes in practice, thus giving the register a membership of up-to-date practitioners (UKCC, 1990). There has been little debate on how to test the clinical skills of those on the register and it could be argued that clinical supervision might provide some confidence in their clinical competence.

It is interesting to note that family doctors are obliged to attend periodic training days but receive payment for attending in-service education and it would be encouraging to see a similar opportunity in nursing.

5. Clinical supervision requires time and energy and is not an incidental event.
The British Association for Counselling have made recommendations that their recognized supervisors will have 'an on-going arrangement for consultation and supervision'. This implies that there is a specific time commitment to clinical supervision and that those doing it are available and in practice. It is evident that those carrying out clinical supervision in nursing will need to be familiar with, and expert in, clinical practice. There are some so-called 'clinical manager' positions which are held by nurses who have not practised for a considerable period and their ability to give clinical supervision must be questionable. Happily this is not generally the case and the level of clinical expertise available is often of the highest quality.

For clinical supervision to gain a foothold in nursing, sufficient time will be needed to conduct supervision sessions within the working day. As productivity conscious managers strive for constantly improved performance this may be hard to establish.

## EVIDENCE OF CHANGE

There is some clear evidence that nurses are beginning to think about clinical supervision. The English National Board for Nurses, Midwives and Health Visitors (1989) has made public its concern in these matters and commissioned a research project with the expressed aim of examining 'The relationships between teaching, support, supervision and role modelling for students in clinical areas within the context of Project 2000 courses'.

Work to prepare the profession for Project 2000 has raised new debates in nursing literature and a discussion is emerging on the blur between the roles of 'preceptor', 'mentor' and other kinds of supervisor (Morris *et al.*, 1988).

Problems have been identified with the allocation of students to mentors, workload and commitment to the role (Leonard and Jowett, 1990; Braken and Davies, 1989) and there is some evidence to suggest that role preparation has not resolved these difficulties. It may be that in those areas where primary nursing has been introduced mentorship and supervision are better facilitated. Pearson (1988), reporting his work in Oxford, shows the importance of placing a value upon dynamic relationships. Interesting exploratory work by Lidbetter (1990) suggests that students place a high value on supervisors and mentors. She suggests that one of the most significant findings of her study on the satisfaction of students working in primary nursing and team nursing was 'the contribution made by students' mentors'. Moreover students believed their mentors taught them theory and practice more often.

It may take time to absorb the principles of clinical supervision into nursing and its day-to-day activities. It is perhaps necessary to look at some of the theoretical paradigms which underpin clinical supervision and how a working model for nursing might be culled from these paradigms and the practices already to be found in nursing itself, for the profession is not without a track record in these matters. What is essential is that the good work already to be found in nursing is not abandoned in search of a new 'holy grail'. As will be seen by the reader, this book is not only a source of ideas from the many specialties in nursing but also a declaration of good practices.

## REFERENCES

Braken, E. and Davies, J. (1989) The implications of mentorship in nursing career development, *Senior Nurse*, 9(5), 5 May, 15–16.

Brammer, L. (1979) *The Helping Relationship*, Prentice Hall, New York.

Burnard, P. (1988) Mentors: A supporting act, *Nursing Times*, 16 Nov., 84(46), 27–8.

Burnard, P. (1989) The role of mentor, *Journal of District Nursing*, 8(3), 8–17.

Butterworth, C. A. (1990) The nurse practitioner in the United Kingdom. Paper given to the National Organization of Nurse Practitioner Faculty, University of Texas, Galveston.

Copp, G. (1988) The reality behind stress, *Nursing Times*, 9 Nov., 84(45), 50–3.

Cox, T. (1978) *Stress*, Macmillan, New York.

Darling, L. A. (1984) What do nurses want in a Mentor? *Journal of Nursing Administration*, Oct., 14(10), 42–44.

Department of Health (1989) Report of the Advisory Group on Nurse Prescribing (Crown Report), HMSO, London.

English National Board for Nurses, Midwives and Health Visitors (ENB) (July

1989) Preparation of Teachers, Practitioner/Teachers, Mentors and Supervisors in the Context of Project 2000.

Freudenberger, H. J. (1975) The staff burn-out syndrome, *Psychotherapy: Theory, Research and Practice*, **12**, 73–82.

Hill, J. (1989) Supervision in the caring professions: A literature review, *Community Psychiatric Nursing Journal*, Oct., **9**(5), 9–15.

Jarvis, P. and Gibson, S. (1985) *The Teacher Practitioner in Nursing, Midwifery and Health Visiting*, Croom Helm, London.

Leonard, A. and Jowett, S. (1990) *Project 2000 Charting the Course*, National Foundation for Education Research.

Lidbetter, J. (1990) A better way to learn? *Nursing Times*, 18 July, **86**(29), 61–4.

McCarthy, P. (1985) Burnout in psychiatric nursing, *Journal of Advanced Nursing*, **10**, 305–10.

Menzies, I. E. P. (1960) *The Functioning of Social Systems as a Defence against Anxiety: a report on a study of the nursing service of a general hospital*, Tavistock Publications, London.

Morris, N., John, G. and Keen, Y. (1988) Mentors: learning the ropes, *Nursing Times*, **84**(46), 24–26.

Northcott, N. (1989) Mentorship in nurse education, *Nursing Standard*, 11 March, **3**(24), 25.

Pearson, A. (1988) *Primary Nursing. Nursing in the Burford and Oxford Nursing Development Units*, Croom Helm, London.

Pembrey, S. (1980) *The Ward Sister, Key to Nursing*, RCN Publications, London.

Platt-Koch, L. M. (1986) Clinical supervision for psychiatric nurses, *Journal of Psychological Nursing*, **26**(1), 7–15.

Puetz, B. E. (1985) Learn the ropes from a mentor, *Nursing Success Today*, **2**(6), 11–13.

Rogers, C. (1951) *Client Centred Therapy*, Constable, London.

Royal College of Nursing (1988a) *Boundaries of Nursing: A Policy Statement*, RCN, London.

Royal College of Nursing (1988b) *Specialties in Nursing: A Report of the Working Party Investigating the Development of Specialties within the Nursing Profession*, RCN, London.

Stilwell, B. (1988) Patient attitudes to a highly developed extended role – The Nurse Practitioner. *Recent Advances in Nursing*, **21**, 82–100.

Stockwell, E. (1972) *The Unpopular Patient*, Royal College of Nursing, London.

United Kingdom Central Council for Nursing, Midwifery and Health Visiting (UKCC) (1990) The Report of the Post-Registration Education and Practice Project (PREPP), UKCC, London.

Westheimer, I. J. (1977) *The Practice of Supervision in Social Work*, Ward Lock Educational, London.

Wright, S. G. (1986) *Building and Using a Model of Nursing*, Edward Arnold, London.

# CHAPTER TWO

# The supervisory relationship

## Jean Faugier

In striving to improve their understanding and practice of nursing, nurses have recognized the importance of a supervisory relationship which is outside traditional hierarchical roles. The term 'supervisor' conjures up for nurses ideas of discipline and criticism, and for many of them it is a word with more managerial than clinical connotations. Watts (1987) suggests that

> The generally held conception of supervision is of a lower management activity in which a group of workers is overseen by a supervisor for a variety of reasons such as ensuring timekeeping, processing pay entitlements, regulating rates of work, and monitoring the quality of work according to pre-set standards.

That nurses at all levels, from senior nursing staff to students, require a relationship which focuses primarily on the process and experience of nursing, is something which the profession has been slow to accept. There are of course notable examples of the opposite, both nationally and internationally: nurses in North America have for some time now adopted a more psychodynamic/humanist understanding of the individual and many general and psychiatric nurses in the United States have established supervisory and mentor relationships which focus on these philosophies. In Britain, pockets of psychiatric and general nurses working in specialized or community settings have for some time been acutely aware of the importance of clinical supervision in improving their skills. Barber and Swansberg (1987) describe supervision as

> an interpersonal process in which the skilled practitioner helps a less skilled or experienced practitioner to achieve professional abilities

appropriate to his role, at the same time being offered counsel and support.

In order to develop these relationships which were previously not thought to be essential to good nursing practice, nurses have been forced to adopt models from other disciplines. Whilst there is indeed a wealth of experience and some excellent texts on supervision in areas such as social work, psychotherapy and teaching, it is often only through the adoption of a new philosophical orientation that nurses can obtain experience of these models. Although the impetus for the development of whatever supervision exists within nursing has undoubtedly come from those nurses who have taken that step, it is neither possible nor desirable for all nurses to shift their philosophical orientation from nursing to psychotherapeutic, social or educational models.

In skilled hands, however, such theoretical and practical experience from other disciplines can have a very beneficial effect. The skilled nurse with experience of supervision in psychotherapy, for example, should be capable of selectively adapting psychodynamic supervision for use in nursing situations. Unfortunately, all too often such models are transferred lock, stock and barrel, and as such are experienced as inappropriate and limited, with little reference to the nurse's role.

In those areas where nurses have managed to develop models of excellence in supervision of clinical practice, they may be viewed by colleagues as elitist and removed from the real experience of the 'average nurse'. Nursing has traditionally been intolerant and suspicious of anything which smacks of indulgence, and it can effectively deal with fears of such developments by isolating those practitioners, labelling them as different from the mainstream.

> Supervision in the helping profession has too long been considered an art form reserved only for the master practitioner. (Ivey, 1977)

In the course of this chapter, we hope to provide guidelines to good practice in developing and managing the supervisory relationship in nursing settings.

It behoves us first to examine the nature of the supervisory relationship described by writers from related professions. Without this, we are in danger of re-inventing the wheel, and possibly a wheel of inferior quality.

Almost echoing the developments in nursing in the last few years, Westheimer (1977) was bemoaning the lack of importance attributed to supervision in social work:

> There is much general ignorance about the nature and process of supervision, with its major objective of bringing about an effective

client service. Social workers who find themselves promoted overnight to the position of supervisor receive little help, if any, with their new functions and tasks. Mostly they are not secure enough to declare their needs for further education in this sphere, afraid of being thought incompetent.

Since the post-Seebohm (1968) days in which Westheimer was writing, further reorganizations of social work have served to underline the importance of the supervisor's role and the need for its further development. The arrival of scores of newly trained social workers in inner city areas with inadequate levels of casework supervision continues to be a grave cause for concern to the profession and society, often only being revealed in a somewhat dramatic manner when a case goes tragically wrong for the want of experienced input to case supervision. However, some outstanding work on supervision has been achieved in the field of social work by such theorists as Kadushin (1976) and Pettes (1979), whose pioneering efforts have done much to make casework supervision an accepted and expected part of practice for social workers of all grades.

The other major contribution to our understanding of the nature of supervisory practice has come from psychotherapy. Drawing largely on the experience of clinical supervision as undertaken in psychoanalysis, the major emphasis here is a study of the interactive and communications systems contained in the therapist–client relationship and the therapist–supervisor relationship. This form of clinical supervision is often very structured and involves a complicated network of motivations revealed in the triadic dimensions of the supervisory relationship. Inevitably, a treatment orientation such as psychoanalysis, which concentrates on working with the unconscious life of the patient, will essentially reflect such an orientation in the supervisory process. Long-term treatment of patients over many years is mirrored by similar long-term relationships between supervisors and supervisees in which the defences and resistances of the trainee therapist are as interesting to the supervisor as those of the patient, and often more so, as they frequently represent evidence of transference relationships developing in the therapeutic process. Wolberg (1988) writes:

> It is almost inevitable that psychotherapists will be influenced by unconscious processes in their patients. Patients who have incorporated parental messages and repudiated their presence may through projective identification accuse the therapist of the very impulses which they deny in themselves. More insidiously, the projections may not be direct, but the therapist will become aware of them through countertransference, perhaps reflected in dreams or fantasies.

The understanding of these processes is absolutely vital to the safe practice of psychotherapy, and writers such as Langs (1979) point out that a failure to recognize such phenomena through the medium of supervision can lead to destructive acting out behaviour by the therapist typified by feelings of aggression or smothering overprotectiveness. One of the prime duties of the supervisor is to assist the supervisee to recognize such communications when they occur and to work through them via the medium of the supervisory relationship rather than the therapeutic one. This model of supervisory practice works within strict contractual boundaries over lengthy periods of training, and whilst such intensive supervision is highly desirable for those wishing to work as psychotherapists, it is not appropriate for those who have shorter-term, less intensive, therapeutic relationships. Analysts such as Balint (1957), Malan (1975) and Hobson (1985) have clearly recognized this shortcoming and have adapted psychodynamic models to shorter-term therapeutic work.

These models, which, like all psychodynamic work, are based on the requirement of good quality supervision, have been used successfully with general practitioners, nurses and social workers in particular.

## THE SUPERVISORY RELATIONSHIP IN PSYCHOTHERAPY

Describing the manner in which various influences have shaped the view of supervision in psychotherapy, Wolberg (1988) claims that skilled supervisors must deftly weave their way through the sometimes very disparate needs of the supervisees, patients and institutions, until they can somehow fuse the various elements into a serviceable amalgam. Whilst not discounting the earlier influences of psychoanalysis, supervision in psychotherapy is currently moving towards a more eclectic model whose primary function is not 'therapy' for the supervisee, but which concentrates instead on the educational and evaluative elements of the supervisory situation.

Increasingly, supervision is being viewed as an essential educational process vital to the acquisition of effective therapeutic skills, central to professional growth. Supervision is about the overall functioning of the therapist in the clinical situation, and this is unlikely to be assessed by concentrating solely on the subconscious of the trainee. It is however unlikely to be assessed fully should this be ignored. In order to achieve this balance in therapeutic practice, it may be necessary to bring to the supervisees's attention that they have failed to live up to therapeutic potential, either due to lack of knowledge or skill, or because of unresolved neurotic character traits which impinge on the relationship with patient or supervisor.

When identifying personal problems in the supervisee, it is not the role of the supervisor to change the emphasis from supervision to therapy, but to raise awareness in the hope that the supervisee will be encouraged to undertake personal therapy to resolve such issues. The primary task of supervision is to assist supervisees in gaining knowledge that is lacking, helping them in establishing and maintaining the therapeutic relationship, overcoming resistance to learning, and in undertaking an evaluation of their skills and capacities for the purpose of professional development. By providing a 'safe environment', the supervisor in psychotherapy can help the supervisee to make great strides in theoretical understanding, therapeutic aptitudes, and abilities to form and sustain relationships with both patients and supervisors.

## THE SUPERVISORY RELATIONSHIP IN SOCIAL WORK

In attempting to prioritize the requirements of the supervisor's role in social work practice, Westheimer (1977) places the emphasis on the educational elements:

> Supervision is an individual method of learning further in the performance of a responsible job. To help people learn, to ask questions in a way which leads to well considered and appropriate decisions, calls for theoretical knowledge, practical skills, and experience as a competent social worker.

Westheimer goes on to attempt to delineate the requirements of the supervisor in furthering knowledge: the possession and consolidation of knowledge, teaching skill, empathy for clients and colleagues, enjoyment in the development of others, familiarity with agency structure, an ability to regulate emotional pressures, appropriate use of authority, and a willingness to develop. Clearly supervision is not a task for those lacking in either experience or insight.

Middleman and Rhodes (1985) point out that the most frequently expressed desire of workers in the field, as is so often the case in nursing, relates to the areas of increased autonomy and esteem in respect of their individual practice. In an attempt to facilitate such developments, they postulate nine areas of emphasis for the would-be social work supervisor:

1. the personal and interpersonal aspects of supervision;
2. encouraging self-acceptance;
3. giving feedback;
4. encouraging interpersonal regard, the development of trust, caring and interdependence;

5.  managing tension;
6.  helping the supervisee deal with uncertainties, and fostering clinical autonomy;
7.  facilitating the recognition of clinical boundaries and limitations in skill and competence;
8.  enhancing morale in order to inspire and motivate towards excellence;
9.  helping supervisees recognize the service delivery functions of their role, in order to respond to the client in conformity with the ethical bases and values of the profession.

## LESSONS FOR NURSING

There can be little doubt that a close examination of the functions of the supervisor and the nature of the supervisory relationship would prove useful to nursing. However, the rather piecemeal nature of its development has resulted in a fragmented understanding within the nursing profession of the importance of supervision in clinical practice. Frequently, one sees 'the need for supervision' tacked on to the end of a training programme or a description of a nursing model as if it is something which simply happens. It would seem that our colleagues from social work and psychotherapy learned some time ago that unless a thorough examination of what is meant by clinical supervision is undertaken, time set aside for it to happen, and an outline of the duties and requirements of the supervisor clearly made, it is likely to remain an unfulfilled demand repeated at every opportunity by clinical workers.

In the past decade, much has been written on the need for supervision in nursing but comparatively little has been written on effective techniques, or on the roles and requirements within the supervisory relationship. Recently there have been exciting developments in the profession which have involved the integration of previously discrete clinical orientations. Behaviourists are now seen in open dialogue with psychodynamic colleagues, counselling coexists alongside 'high-tech' approaches, such as invasive surgery and investigation; the influence of complementary therapies on the practice of a great many nurses is now an established fact. Supervision of such diverse clinical practice must itself take an eclectic framework if it is to contain the all-important elements of education and support whilst resisting the temptation to become too rigid and dogmatic. The need pragmatically to blend clinical models is common even in areas of clinical practice which claim a strong adherence to one philosophical position. Day-to-day experience with patients and clients underlines the need for such flexibility, if we are to avoid imposing our 'favourite' approach to treatment and care upon them inappropriately.

A similar approach has been developed by Halgin (1986) to the supervisory relationship:

> The realm of individual supervision is an optimal format within which to communicate to trainees the excitement of the growing trend to therapeutic integration. Not only can teachers convey to supervisees the utility of therapeutic integration, but they have the invaluable opportunity to demonstrate it to them within the context of the supervisory relationship.

Just as one would expect the nurse to have the ability selectively to blend various clinical approaches in response to the patients' needs, the supervisor should be able to demonstrate such an ability during clinical supervision. Examples from psychodynamic theory, behavioural theory, interpersonal humanistic theories, biological theories and sociological theories all have a major contribution to make to a working model of clinical supervision for nurses.

## THE GROWTH AND SUPPORT MODEL OF THE SUPERVISORY RELATIONSHIP

In an attempt to provide some guidelines to the characteristics of the supervisory relationship which are essential to good practice, we offer here one particular way of looking at the various elements.

The role of the supervisor is to facilitate **growth** both educationally and personally in the supervisee, whilst providing essential **support** to their developing clinical autonomy. In order to achieve this, the supervisor must be aware of elements of the relationship for which they are responsible.

### Generosity

This is an essential requirement in a supervisor or mentor, and does not simply refer to supplying the coffee during the supervision session, although the provision of such seemingly unimportant items can add significantly to the atmosphere and experience of supervision. In particular, supervisors will need to be generous with their time, which is often precious and in short supply, especially to the experienced trained nurse responsible for the well-being of patients as well as colleagues. Instructions such as 'Let's see if we can find some time tomorrow, shall we?', or 'Make sure you bring that issue up when I am on duty next', can be extremely discouraging to supervisees who may fear that they will be considered a nuisance and inadequate if they request supervision.

This inability to place clinical supervision in a position of priority means that all other activities, such as answering the telephone, dealing with enquiries and with medical staff, attending to administration, etc., are always eating into the time needed for supervision.

It is also important that the supervisor displays a generosity of spirit. Supervision with someone who finds it difficult to give either intellectually or emotionally within the supervisory relationship will be unsuccessful in providing the all-important inspiration which can only arise truly from a well managed transference relationship. Significantly too, supervision with an absence of generosity can be a very punitive experience, leaving the supervisee confused and angry.

## Rewarding

Development and effort deserve to be rewarded. A supervisee will frequently display marked ability in certain areas at an exceptionally high level. It is the duty of the mature supervisor (the term is used with no reference to age, but implies that the supervisor has been through the processes now being experienced by the supervisee, and has derived some insight from the journey) to further such development by rewarding in the form of praise and encouragement. It is not appropriate for any supervisor or mentor to use the supervisory relationship to deal with unresolved feelings of inadequacy or insecurity. Self-awareness is therefore a pre-requisite for selection as a supervisor and the institution or service should ensure that such training is undertaken prior to working in a responsible position as a supervisor. Moreover, such self-awareness should of course be ongoing, and supervisors themselves should have access to either personal or group supervision in order to facilitate this process. Casement (1985) emphasizes this process of self-development contained within the supervisor's role:

> Just as we can see our own errors more clearly in others, so too in supervising others. Here there are endless opportunities for therapists to re-examine their own work, when looking closely at the work of the person being supervised. Not infrequently, supervisors will be seeing reflections of their own difficulties with technique. We do not always do as we teach others to do, but we can learn a lot by trying.

Although writing about psychotherapy, Bion (1975) coined the term which perhaps exemplifies this process of continued self-awareness development necessary in the supervisor, when he claimed we should always be in a state of **becoming**. Those nurses who, upon qualifying, feel that they know all they need to know, not only about nursing but also about themselves, should never be given the opportunity to stunt the growth of others through the medium of supervision.

## Openness

In the course of supervising a process as complex and demanding as nursing, difficult and awkward times will frequently occur. The real nature of our human existence, characterized by uncertainty, tension, confusion, irritation and anger, is vividly displayed when illness occurs, either in ourselves or those we care for. The problems which nurses have in coping with this tapestry of emotional and physical responses can be and are often mirrored in the supervisory process. Problems and tensions which arise between supervisor and supervisee can in effect often turn out to be the very essence of the learning experience, allowing the supervisee to give voice to something which would otherwise remain a worrying feeling. The authors have frequently been in the position of 'not knowing' in the supervision of others. This is particularly true when the material presented for supervision is very distressing or disturbing, or the physical condition of the patient is life threatening, disabling or disfiguring.

The tradition in nursing is for the person in the educational role such as the clinical supervisor to provide the answers, to be all-knowing. And yet the most important learning experience the supervisor can provide is openness to feelings and experience, i.e. simply being able to stay with the feelings of the supervisee and therefore vicariously with the patient. The need to fill voids and cover gaps by intervention has always been nursing's way of dealing with anxiety, and it is important for the supervisor not to become an example of this.

The **parallel process**, identified by Eckstein and Wallenstein (1958), refers to the analogy between the experience of the patient–supervisee relationship and that of the supervisor/supervisee. For example, a nurse who is angry with the world and medical science for failing to help a young male patient dying with HIV, angry with the young man himself for leaving her when she is now so fond of him, and angry with herself for also not being able to be the 'perfect nurse' who would avoid such feelings, will almost certainly express some of these feelings at some stage in supervision in the form of overt or covert anger and hostility towards the supervisor whom she perhaps perceives as failing to keep her protected from these painful emotions. It is in these difficult times that much of the real learning about nursing will take place, by supervisors displaying an ability to remain open to such parallel processes and use them to gain a greater understanding of all concerned, including themselves. At times like this, when feelings are on the surface, it will help the supervisor to remember the old maxim that 'anyone can hold the helm when the sea is calm'.

## Willingness to learn

Nursing organization, infested as it is with the constraints of hierarchy, can appear to be a system loaded against the development of continued learning. Sensitivity to position and seniority are handicaps which hamper the recognition of personal limitations and the ability to listen to others. This threat of losing position or 'face' before junior or untrained members of staff arises from a serious misconception endemic in nursing: the belief that one can ever know all there is to know even about one's own role and that such knowledge is static. As George Bernard Shaw pointed out in 'Major Barbara': 'You have learned something, that always feels as though you have lost something'. How many of us have felt that gradual loss of certainty in our careers as we have moved from the completion of training to face the ambiguity at the heart of our profession?

Supervisors who fail to maintain an ability to continue learning throughout their careers are denying the very dynamic nature of nursing, and will be in constant fear of being engulfed by the oncoming tide of development represented by the person of their supervisees.

## Thoughtful and thought provoking

The participants in the supervisory process invariably bring to the situation their own agenda. The supervisees are interested in learning 'nursing' or some special related skill, in order to gain a qualification or obtain promotion. The supervisor on the other hand wishes to demonstrate competence as a senior clinical nurse whilst providing an environment in which supervisees can safely grow in terms of skill and intellect. The hospital, institution or service wishes to ensure that the patient receives a certain standard of nursing care, and sees supervision as one way of ensuring this. The many and various aims and aspirations placed upon the supervisory process can have the effect of diverting it from one of its two major roles, the **educative function**. The provision of adequate learning for supervisees presupposes an ability to present material in a way which will enable them to make the necessary cognitive links. Wolberg (1988) uses a particularly vivid example to draw attention to this need to stimulate intellectual understanding in supervisees:

A professional coach who sends his or her players out to complete a number of practice games, with instructions on what to do, and who asks them to provide a verbal report at intervals of how they played and what they intended to do next, would probably last no more than one season. What is lacking is a systematic critique of actual performances as observed by peers and supervisors.

The 'coach', then, must lead from the front, must have access to actual data in the form of observations, recordings, or video material, and must seek to stimulate thought by offering informed theory-based links to the practice problems of the supervisee. All this of course demands a knowledge base on the part of the supervisor.

## Humanity

McFarlane (1982) described nursing as the **art of caring**. By its very nature, nursing is a profession touched by the sorrows and joys of mankind in a very special way. The privileged position of being the person who provides intimate physical care to people in their times of greatest need and dependence is the basis of all good nursing. In order to fulfil our function to a high standard and retain the inherent dignity of those for whom we care, we must have within ourselves, and instil in those we supervise, a sense of that dignity. Supervisors will reflect this by the way they set the tone for the discussion of patients and their problems, and accept human frailties. Humour is not out of place in supervision however; human beings are frequently comical characters. Perhaps the best example of supervisors' humanity is their ability to treat supervisees as worthy human beings in whose development they are privileged to be involved.

## Sensitivity

A supervision session is a live encounter in the 'here and now' between two human beings. It is inevitable that each person brings to that encounter their uniqueness as an individual. It is also inevitable that each of the participants brings with them issues which are currently important for them outside of that situation. Sensitivity to personal and interpersonal work barriers is a crucial feature of effective supervision. Nursing has traditionally been a hierarchical and organizationally bureaucratic profession, noted for its tendency to over-emphasize the technical and organizational at the expense of the personal and interpersonal. A clear reflection of this tendency is seen in the reinforcing and rewarding of impersonality in relationships, defined as 'professionalism', the emphasis in nursing on behavioural strategies as 'separate problems', and the compartmentalization of task allocation.

Such an approach results in a corresponding lack of concern for the whole person; it also works against the development of confident nurses with high personal regard for themselves and others. A feeling that one is appreciated, needed and a sense that one's work is progressing along valued lines are all essential aspects of producing self-acceptance in nursing. Frequently a supervisee will bring to supervision what they believe sincerely to be their best effort. Sometimes this best effort will have failed to produce anything but a disappointing outcome, or else an intervention will be viewed too optimistically by the supervisee. Middleman and Rhodes (1985) point out that, in such circumstances, it is too easy to give blanket commonsense responses to the frustrations and disappointments of the supervisee, when what is needed are 'uncommon-sense' responses: as a supervisor, it is necessary to give a response which reflects a sensitive appreciation of the work which has been put in, and the subsequent feelings of failure and guilt when the supervisee realizes that much of the effort may have been misguided, or has failed to show the hoped for results. This ability to value the nurse and her efforts can lead to the supervision session being used effectively for the purpose of education, i.e. exploring all the alternative strategies and interventions possible in the examined clinical situation.

## Uncompromising

The dictionary definition of 'uncompromising' is 'not allowing or seeking compromise', 'unyielding or stubborn'. At first glance, this hardly seems a feature one would wish to include in a 'progressive' model of nursing supervision. And yet an uncompromising rigour is one of the most vital contributions an effective supervisor can bring to the overall process. The practice of nursing cannot be open to any compromise in the standards of care for individual patients, and this should be reflected in the supervisory process. By making use of probing casework, peer group assessment, supervisor observation and the interpretation of individual presentations, the supervisor can maintain an atmosphere in which warmth and understanding go hand-in-hand with clinical and intellectual rigour. In addition, supervisors must establish an atmosphere of uncompromising confidentiality, trust and professionalism. These issues, particularly that of the maintenance of therapeutic boundaries, can be demonstrated to the supervisee as part of the relationship within supervision, which may then be applied to other relationships outside, with patients and staff in the clinical setting.

The most difficult task of supervision is often the acknowledgement of problems 'seated' in oneself, and the need for more awareness of such issues. Supervisees sometimes employ classic 'approach avoidance' mechanisms in order to deal with such difficulties, and an uncompromising rigour is once again needed to ensure that supervisees make the necessary links not only with theory and practice, but also with their own feelings.

## Personal

Supervision of clinical practice may be carried out in a great number of both settings and styles. It will nevertheless have some essentially common features: it should, by definition, centre on the clinical work of nursing, the central focus of which is the relationship—the vehicle of nursing; additionally, it will commonly have an educational function and should therefore seek to increase self-awareness on the part of the supervisee.

Despite these common elements, however, it remains a personal experience, and should not be subjected to any unnecessary structure. Each individual supervisor or mentor will display individual personal styles, and it is important to consider and give due merit to this individuality when asking nurses to choose a supervisor. Sadly, the move to mentorship and clinical supervision in nursing has been marked in too many cases by a lack of understanding of the personal nature of the supervisory relationship, which has only contributed to devaluing the process and reducing its effectiveness in improving practice. The all pervading notion that 'any nurse can nurse any patient' is transposed lock, stock and barrel to supervision and becomes 'any supervisor can supervise any supervisee'. This is patently not the case, and simply serves to perpetuate the celebration of the impersonal which runs throughout our development as a profession.

## Practical

Any supervision session in which a nurse does not acquire new skills in delivery of care, even if she feels more self-aware, constitutes a failure. Nursing is a practically based profession. Care is delivered not only through emotional regard and psychological input, but also by the very practical measures which are vital to the patients' well-being as well as representing a tangible expression of care. The educational process of supervision must therefore focus on practice and its improvement.

The development of **knowledge**, **attitudes** and **skills** in nursing often places too little emphasis on the latter. In a profession that for decades has been plagued by a pragmatic approach to the 'how' of practice with little regard for the 'what' and the 'why', we have recently, and somewhat self-consciously, reversed the coin in an attempt to understand theoretical and attitudinal issues in greater depth. Whilst this is extremely important, it carries along with it the danger of ignoring the practical issues of the 'how', with the result that clinical practice can, and does, suffer. The effective supervisor must guard against an over-intellectual, woolly approach to essentially practical interventions; neither must he/she assume that the supervisee will intuitively know 'how' to do 'what'. Clinical supervisors in nursing are provided with a wonderful opportunity in providing 'skills modelling' training. An example of this is provided by Brammer and Wassmer (1979) in their description of supervising trainee counsellors. In pointing to the dearth of outcome measures in counselling training, they plead the case for more focus on the 'behaviours' of supervisees as well as on knowledge and attitudes.

## Orientation

As Wolberg (1988) points out, important and often irreconcilable differences occur in the theoretical background and orientation of the supervisor and the supervisee. Such differences may express themselves in nursing in any of the following ways:

1. The relative weight placed on biological as opposed to psychological and social factors in the genesis of a patient's problems.
2. The value of particular forms of intervention, particularly when such intervention may be seen as invasive and distressing for the patient.
3. The degree of stress which is placed on personality or character issues in determining individual behaviour.
4. Differences in prioritization of long-term and short-term nursing objectives.

The most effective supervision of nursing practice is the one which shows respect for the ideas and opinions of others. However, it is also the role of the supervisor to guide the supervisee to a position of recognizing when extreme opinions are in conflict with the needs of the patient and the delivery of appropriate nursing care. Goal setting may assist in producing a discussion and resolution of any differences and may help both parties in seeing that they have generally more to agree about than to disagree. Supervisees may have to accept that a very modest treatment goal is not necessarily a negation of deeply held principles, but simply a more realistic means of caring for the patient in the 'here and now'.

Important in this process of negotiation between supervisor and supervisee is effective communication. Matters which may seem like 'affaires d'état' may frequently be due to the absence of a mutual language and a lack of listening to the latent content of what is being said.

For the most part, sensitive handling can resolve these issues to the benefit of all concerned. There are however some occasions when it becomes necessary to acknowledge that fundamental differences in orientation do exist, and that the nurse concerned should seek supervision from someone more in tune with the way she interprets nursing practice. Nursing is a 'broad church', and there should be room for everyone, especially as there are different roads to the same end product.

## Relationship

The supervisor's role is to assist the supervisee to apply theoretical knowledge, appropriate attitudes and the art of therapeutic communication to the treatment of patients. This is done primarily through the medium of the supervisory relationship:

> In supervision, the nurse gains theoretical knowledge but also learns to make new and fuller use of the self. (Platt-Koch, 1986)

This emphasis on self-awareness issues in supervision can sometimes serve to blur the boundaries, and supervisors may find themselves conducting a personal therapy rather than a supervision session.

Although supervision and psychotherapy are both helping processes, they differ significantly in their primary purpose and focus. Psychotherapy is about helping people to deal with inner conflicts and neurotic symptomatology. Supervision is about helping the nurse to increase her working skills more effectively with patients. Whilst this certainly involves more self-awareness, and the supervisor is involved in facilitating personal growth, the distinction between the therapeutic and supervisory relationship should be maintained. Platt-Koch (1986) refers to this similarity with psychotherapy and the **parallel process** which should be fostered but not exploited.

> Again there is a parallel to psychotherapy, in which the patient is helped to develop awareness of how thoughts and feelings affect behaviour. The patient can then make choices about how to live.

The alliance between supervisor and supervisee is analogous to the therapeutic alliance defined as the bond of trust between nurse and patient which is necessary for the practice of high quality nursing. By exploiting the emphasis on self-awareness issues in supervision, the supervisee may attempt to receive 'therapy' from the supervisor, thereby diverting the sessions into a situation where personal needs are the centre of attention. Similarly, supervisors may wish to demonstrate their own understanding of the human psyche and may be guilty of over-analysing the responses of the supervisee, which often leads to resentment and anger. All these relationship 'traps' do nothing to serve the real purpose of supervision, which is the promoting of learning about nursing, including some personal growth content.

Change is a difficult process for all of us, and at times the relationship in supervision can become 'stuck' in resistance to change which can take many forms, all usually related to difficulties experienced in the clinical situation with patients. Feeling comfortable with the idea of sharing one's work and feelings about it with a supervisor can also give rise to understandable sentiments of anxiety. Peplau (1957) contends that a certain optimum level of anxiety in the supervisory relationship is healthy and vitally necessary for any change or learning to take place. However, when these anxiety levels become too high, they must be addressed as they tend to interfere with learning and with the conduct of the supervision session. A common fantasy of supervisees is what might be termed the 'glass head syndrome' in which they come to believe early in a supervisory relationship that the more experienced, more qualified supervisor has the ability to know what is in their heads without them saying anything. That anxiety provoking situation, if suspected, should be talked through. For Haller (1976), quality supervision depends on this ability of both parties to discuss the relationship itself when a problem prevents understanding and growth. Platt-Koch (1986) sums up the relationship of supervision thus:

> Despite occasional problems, supervision should feel like a safe place for the nurse. Concomitantly, the supervisor should feel pleasure in nurturing a younger or less experienced clinician.

### Trust

Although this comes last in our description of the supervisory relationship, without trust there is no relationship. The supervisee, feeling exposed and without defences, must have absolute trust in the supervisor to keep them 'safe'. Reliability and consistency in word and action are important in providing an atmosphere in which the supervisee feels that the supervisor may be depended upon, whether this applies to commitments made for sessions or any other form of assistance. Essentially, one is aiming to provide what Rogerians describe as **unconditional positive regard** in the work situation. This means providing an atmosphere in which deficits in knowledge, attitudes or skills may be explored without being interpreted as a (negative) comment on the supervisee personally.

Closely linked to the development of such a climate is the sense of caring conveyed to supervisees by the time commitment and the energy invested on their behalf. Genuineness cannot be faked; the rule is: if you don't really care about the development of other nurses and nursing, don't become a supervisor, as it will only prove a persecutory relationship for those in your charge. Discussing trust in therapy, Dryden (1987) claims that one of our biggest problems lies in trusting ourselves:

> The person centred approach is based on the belief that the human organism is trustworthy and that we have within us the necessary wisdom and resources for our development to full human-ness. And yet, how difficult it seems to be for those of us who are therapists to trust the truth of this assertion when we ourselves are the organism in question and when that organism is prompting in us a loving and spontaneous response to another person. Clearly, it is right and proper that we should be cautious for we know our capacity for self deception can be great.

In affirming the supervisee's strengths, and recognizing the emotional demands of the nursing situation, the supervisor can make inroads into helping supervisees trust themselves and therefore others. As Middleman and Rhodes point out: 'In essence, by word and by deed, the supervisor contributes to the nurse's self acceptance and confirmation'.

The establishment of trust also requires a high level of professionalism in the operation of supervisory boundaries. Supervision can place both parties in a strong transference situation. The intimate discussion of clinical and personal issues can, and should, have the effect of producing closeness between supervisor and supervisee. Some inexperienced nurses may misinterpret the interest and concern of the supervisor or may openly express feelings of love and sexual attraction. These can be very difficult tests of trust and understanding for the sensitive supervisor who, whilst insisting on the retention of strictly professional boundaries, has no desire to hurt or humiliate the supervisee. The important learning experience for the latter is that sexual issues so often hidden in nursing can be discussed and the outcome remain positive. Trusting a supervisor with very intimate feelings without being overwhelmed by negative emotions can be an important learning experience. In the world of nursing, where we so often seem to pretend that gender and sexuality do not exist, it can come as a pleasant surprise to find out that a supervisor has human feelings.

In this chapter, we have attempted to provide a framework on which to base the supervisory relationship. By reference to a guide, such as the growth and support model, supervisors can ensure that all the essential elements of the relationship are given adequate emphasis. However, in presenting the model, we do not wish to imply that there is only one way of providing structure to the supervisory process. Supervision is, as we have stated, a personal as well as a professional experience, and it is precisely this human element which allows for the great breadth and variety of approach.

## REFERENCES

Balint, M. (1957) *The Doctor, His Patient, and the Illness*, Int. University Press, New York.

Barber and Swansberg (1987) Skills in supervision. *Nursing Times*, 1–4. 1. 87.

Bion, W. R. (1975) *Brazilian Lectures*, 1. Imago Editora, Rio de Janeiro.

Brammer, L. M. and Wassmer, A. C. (1979) Supervision in counselling and psychotherapy, in *Supervision of Applied Training* (Ed. D. J. Kurpius *et al.*) Greenwood Press, London.

Burnard, P. (1988) Mentors: A supporting act *Nursing Times*, **83**(2), 14–20.

Casement, P. (1985) *On Learning from the Patient*, Tavistock, London.

Darling, L. A. W. (1984) What do nurses want in a mentor. *Journal of Nursing Administration*, **14**(10), 42–4.

Dryden, W. (1987) *Key Cases in Psychotherapy*, Croom Helm, London.

Eckstein, R. and Wallenstein, R. S. (1958) *The Teaching and Learning of Psychotherapy*, Basic Books, New York.

Halgin, R. P. (1986) Pragmatic blending of clinical model in the supervision relationship, *The Clinical Supervisor*, **3** (Winter 85–86), 23–46.

Haller, L. L. (1976) Clinical psychiatric supervision. Process and problems. A method of teaching psychiatric concepts in nursing education. *Perspectives in Psychiatric Care*, **14**, 115–29.

Hobson, R. (1985) *Forms of Feeling: The Heart of Psychotherapy*, Tavistock, London.

Ivey, A. (1977) Foreword in *Supervision of Applied Training. A Comparative Review*, Kurpius, D. J. *et al.* Greenwood Press, London.

Kadushin, A. (1976) *Supervision in Social Work*, Columbia Press, New York.

Langs, R. (1979) *The Supervisory Experience*, Aronson, New York.

Malan, D. H. (1975) *A Study of Brief Psychotherapy*, Plenum Rosetta, New York.

McCarthy, P. (1985) Burnout in psychiatric nursing. *Journal of Advanced Nursing*, **10**, 305–10.

McFarlane, J. (1982) A charter for caring. *Journal of Advanced Nursing*.

Middleman, R. and Rhodes, G. (1985) *Competent Supervision: Making Imaginative Judgements*, Prentice-Hall, New Jersey.

Peplau, H. E. (1957) What is experiential teaching? *American Journal of Nursing*, 884–6.

Pettes, D. E. (1979) *Staff and Student Supervision: A staff centred approach*, Allen and Unwin, London.

Platt-Koch, L. M. (1986) Clinical supervision for psychiatric nurses. *Journal of Psycho-social Nursing*, January, **26**(1).

Seebohm, F. (1968) *Report of Committee on Local Authority and Personal and Social Services*, HMSO, London.

Watt, G. (1987) *Clinical Supervision in Community Psychiatric Nursing*, Unpublished report, Leeds University.

Westheimer, I. (1977) *The Practice of Supervision in Social Work. A guide for supervisors*, Ward Lock Educational, London.

Wolberg, L. R. (1988) *The Teaching of Psychotherapy*. 4th edn, Part 2. Grune and Stratton, New York.

# CHAPTER THREE

# The therapeutic use of self

## David Woods

### INTRODUCTION

Peter was a nurse working in a hospice. He had worked there for four years and was proud that no other member of staff had worked in the unit for as long and with as little time off for sickness as he had. He had seen other members of staff come and stay for a year or two and leave to work in other branches of nursing. He had supported and cared for a great many patients and had helped them to die with dignity.

In one of the hospice unit's weekly staff support groups he became very upset and disturbed one day and described a recurring dream that he had almost every night. The dream made him feel frightened and anxious for his future. He could not make sense of it and brought it to the group because he was at the end of his tether. This was unusual for Peter, because although he didn't openly scorn the group he didn't think he needed it. In his recurrent dream he was walking down a corridor with doors on either side. He felt compelled to go into each room and in each room lying in bed dying was a member of his own family, reaching out to him for help. He described feeling that he wanted to kill them and as he walked towards them to suffocate them he woke up. This left him feeling distressed and uncomfortable and not knowing what the dream meant to him.

When he discussed it in the group one or two members recognized that the dream was more about his work in the hospice than it was a dream about his family. They were able to give him feedback about the way he was apparently able to tolerate the stress and distress of working in the unit. They were able to reflect back to him that he never seemed to be upset on duty when people died. Peter was able to share with them for the first time his anxieties about working in the unit and his increasing personal distress about wanting to distance himself from people who came on to the unit, feeling that if he nursed them they would surely die.

Over the following months Peter was able to talk more openly about the distress of the deaths of so many people on the unit and eventually decided to leave the unit to work in another branch of nursing. He left with a sense of achievement and was looking forward to the future rather than leaving feeling that he could not cope, which is what had prevented him from leaving before.

Jane had been feeling miserable and depressed for a number of months. She had been feeling increasingly unwell and despondent about her life. She was able to identify the beginnings of her feelings of unhappiness and sadness as starting about the time that her daughter, now aged nine months old, was born. She talked over her symptoms and feelings with her general practitioner and they both agreed that her difficult feelings were related to the birth of her child and that she would probably get over it in time. The general practitioner rightly said to her that if she didn't feel much better she must come back and talk things through with him. Jane didn't feel any better. She felt more depressed and upset about her husband feeling that he didn't understand her and that his work was more important in his life than either she or their daughter.

Jane returned to her general practitioner and they talked through what had been happening to her. He was keen that they shouldn't seek a pharmacological solution to her problems and that she needed the opportunity to resolve both her relationship with her husband and her feelings about the birth of her child. They agreed that it might be helpful for Jane to see somebody regularly to work through her feelings. The general practitioner arranged that Jane should see a nurse who was attached to the Health Centre on a weekly basis.

Jane came every week and spent an hour discussing her feelings and her difficulties. The nurse for her part encouraged Jane to express the feelings that she had and helped her to get in touch with her difficulties. As the sessions continued, Jane, for the first time in her life, felt that someone else understood the difficulties that she had and understood the predicament she was in. She eventually decided that her marriage was no longer sustainable. She felt there were so many differences between her and her husband that she could no longer continue. She was worried about having made this decision but was encouraged and supported in her decision by the nurse. The nurse understood and was able to reflect back to Jane that it was difficult but would probably help her more in the long run. After several months of therapy Jane was divorced and finished her therapy, no longer feeling the need to discuss her feelings. The nurse for her part felt that a good job had been done. Jane had taken more responsibility for her life and, with a lot of help, had made an appropriate decision about ending her marriage.

Three months later Jane returned to her general practitioner chronically depressed and unable to function. She felt in danger of physically abusing her child. She felt she had made an enormous mistake in getting divorced and wasn't sure which way to turn next. The general practitioner discussed it in passing with the nurse who had seen Jane for so many months. The nurse remarked, 'I really don't know why it didn't work for her. When I had my baby and got depressed I was in just the same position as her and my divorce was the making of me. I wonder why it wasn't for her?'.

What is important about these two simple illustrations is that the feelings, anxieties, thoughts and expressions of emotion of the two nurses, both acknowledged and unacknowledged, had a bearing and an influence on the quality of the relationship and affected the outcome of the care. Jane presented herself in extreme distress and sought help for that distress. The outcome and apparent resolution of that distress was not what she really wanted. It is possible to hypothesize that the formulation and conceptualization of Jane's difficulties and the understanding of the way to resolve them was largely shaped by the nurse's own personal experience rather than a clear understanding of Jane's position. It is clear that the solution of separation and divorce may have been appropriate for the nurse. It is not so clear that it was appropriate for Jane. It left her feeling angry at herself for taking the advice but also let down and depressed about the position she was in, which she felt was worse than the position she had started with.

In the first illustration, Peter contained his feelings and did not acknowledge they had any importance in the work he was doing. The denial of his own upset and distress at the painful work he was doing overflowed into his life outside of work and caused him great distress. The danger for Peter and his patients, had he not articulated his difficulties, would have been that he increasingly distanced himself from his patients because he was frightened that he would act out his murderous fantasies.

All nursing activity takes place in the context of a human relationship. That relationship may be a brief, concise and contained relationship which may occur with someone attending an accident and emergency department, or it may be a more complex, ongoing relationship between a nurse and a patient over a long period of time in a ward or in the community.

It is important for nurses to recognize and value the uniqueness of this human relationship between people. Whatever branch of nursing is chosen, whether it be the nursing of the physically sick or those who suffer from poor mental health, it is important to acknowledge the feelings, fantasies and experiences that the nurse brings to the relationship.

Everyone has a life history and the way in which we behave and react and, more importantly, interact in our daily lives is moulded and informed by the personal psychological experiences we have had in our lives. When the nurse interacts and communicates with a patient we cannot and should not deny the internal world or the life experiences of the nurse. Nursing is not an impersonal relationship where the patient is reduced to the position of being a powerless child, with the doctor representing the dominant father, and the nurse acting as mother compliantly servicing the family and carrying out father's wishes. Patients are active, thoughtful, reflective, feeling beings with an equal share in the relationship, however vulnerable and fragile their illness leaves them feeling.

If nurses are to maintain and improve the quality of their relationships with their patients they must make greater efforts to enhance the use of their feelings and emotions. This therapeutic use of the self is central to a living dynamic relationship.

Creating and maintaining a relationship which is going to be ultimately helpful to the patient in restoring him to as healthy a position as possible is not something which comes by chance. The reality is that there are more likely to be problems with maintaining that relationship. These problems can perhaps be discussed in three areas.

## ORGANIZATIONAL STRUCTURE

The way in which nurses can function, and the way in which their relationships with their patients develop, must be taken in the context of the organizational structure in which they exist. Undoubtedly the managerial and economic climate in which health care takes place has changed radically over the last five to ten years. There is a high emphasis on managerialism and an increasingly centralized control of health care (Best, 1987), accompanied by an increased emphasis on 'productivity and through put'. The length of stay in hospital is shorter, and community services are increasingly burdened with large numbers of patients who have been discharged perhaps prematurely. Resources are in reality scarcer (Klein, 1985). Demand for health care expenditure has exceeded resource availability (Gamble and Walkland, 1984; DHSS, 1983; Klein, 1985). Nursing in the 1980s saw a major reorganization in 1982, a change in its management system, with the introduction of general management in 1983/4, and the biggest restructuring and reorganization of its nursing services ever in 1988, the effect of which is not over yet. The start of the 1990s brings the reforms of the NHS and community care provision.

At the same time there has been great emphasis placed on quality assurance, personalizing the service and consumer choice. There has been much criticism of the consumer approach to health care, the main critics claiming that the increased emphasis on consumer choice and personal services is little more than a supermarket window dressing.

This climate of increased managerialism and cash limiting of services imposes tremendous stresses on nurses attempting to have an open helpful relationship with their patients. The danger is that many aspects of nursing care are simply impossible to carry out. Constraints on time and external pressures impose impossible demands. In busy acute wards it is quite common for nurses to return from their two days off and not know any of the patients on their ward. The question must seriously be asked, what is this doing to the ability of the nurse to care appropriately and adequately for the patient? It must feel quite impossible at times to pay attention to the psychological meaning of relationships when there are so many external pressures.

Often, general managers and nurse managers are neither equipped nor sufficiently experienced to understand the importance of creating a culture and structure for care which supports and enhances the ability of nurses. In her classic work Isobel Menzies Lyth (1960) was highly critical of the way in which nursing services were organized, and postulated that they were structured to avoid the personal interaction that took place between nurses and patients and that this was designed to avoid the internal anxiety engendered by intimacy of the relationship.

Interestingly, not to say sadly, Menzies Lyth (1988) has recently expressed that although some things have changed she does not really perceive any major differences in present day organization of nursing, and would appear to be critical of the pursuit of professionalization. She argues that nurses require the opportunity to understand their personal feelings, perceptions and anxieties about their work; in a sense more opportunity for tea and talk rather than yet another reorganization and higher professional qualifications.

There are some examples of improvements in the way in which nursing is organized and the way in which nurses conceptualize their work. Attempts have been made to schematize the needs of patients into the nursing process, and at the same time by attempting to use models, nurses have attempted more clearly to understand and identify the patients' needs. Unfortunately, these models and processes often focus on the individual patient and do not attempt to understand interactions in the context of a relationship. There is an almost universal denial that the nurse's actions, feelings and perceptions of the patient are of any importance. This is equally true in psychiatric nursing with its residual emphasis on organic medical models of mental disease.

The world of modern nursing with its processes, models, high technology, efficiency and output is a very difficult place for the nurse who wishes to emphasize the healing process and values the skills of nurturing, caring and compassion.

## OCCUPATIONAL STRESS

Nursing is often a painful business and the pain experienced by nurses in carrying out their day-to-day work often goes unacknowledged, at great personal cost. Several authors (Maslach, 1976; Maslach and Jackson, 1981; Gowler and Perry, 1983) have identified stress as one of the major reasons why nurses fail to function. Parry and Gowler have identified the cruciform effect as being directly related to stress in the caring professions. They describe a situation where conflicting values exert pressures upon professionals. Professionals with a basic mandate to provide a personal service (the basic mandate in the case of nursing is personal care) may find this mandate directly and indirectly challenged by organizational priorities. The organizational priorities require the professional to respond to other considerations. Briefly stated, the cruciform effect occurs where the individual worker is unable internally to resolve the tension between their basic mandate and the priority constructed by the organization. This inability to tolerate the tension results in four coping behaviours.

First, easing: nurses who ease reduce their contact time with patients, spending considerably more time looking after their colleagues, organizing administrative duties, editing books or journals, or acting as nurse consultants.

Secondly, there is freezing: this is basically a denial of the difficulty of the relationship. Freezers close their eyes to the real world and suffering of their patients. They are very careful to select patients who will get better and accept the professional's limited view of care. They tend to be over-cautious and slavishly follow procedures. It is doubtful, though, whether they help many people.

Thirdly, there are the seizers, who avoid patients by embracing new technologies and techniques which enable them to reformulate the complexity of the human being into a series of technical problems. The ultimate expression of seizing may be retreating into research well away from patient contact.

The fourth coping behaviour as a result of internal stress is the process of melting. This complex and ambivalent form of coping involves a dissolving of relationships with more conventional colleagues. Melters are radical nurses who are only too aware of the discomfort of the cruciform effect. They are vociferous in their criticism of easers, freezers and seizers. This method of coping is in direct contrast to freezing and presents itself as a form of inter-professional tension. Melters attempt to resolve the stresses by turning away from conventional one-to-one relationships and try to interact directly with the community. They disown professional skill and status; they however very rarely disown professional salary but nearly always remain on the pay roll of a conservative organization. The dilemma of the melter is rarely resolved.

These descriptions are not intended to be disparaging but more an indication of the complex way in which individuals cope with the stress placed upon them by their painful work.

Menzies, as indicated above, has identified that the very organization of services enables nurses to defend against the anxiety that is generated by their work. This defence is both organizational and personal: organizational in that the structure legislates against the intimacy of nursing relationships developing fully; and personal, because as Menzies points out, if the individual rejects the organizational defence system and continues to use his or her own, there is a risk of rejection from colleagues. In adopting the organizational defence system there will be an increase in anxiety which might result in nurses finding themselves unable to continue. This interface between individuals' feelings and the way in which nursing is organized creates constant pressure for the individual. Menzies Lyth (1988) noted almost 30 years after her original work that wastage rates for nurses in training are not significantly different now from in 1959.

## PROFESSIONALISM

The pursuit of professional status for nurses may well legislate against the creation and maintenance of helpful relationships with patients. Some writers (Doyle, 1979; Illich, 1977; Navarro, 1976; Wilding, 1982) have stated that the pursuit of professional status may compromise the defined aim of the profession and do more for members of the profession than it does for the clients it seeks to serve.

Professionalization of nursing and its consequences require further discussion if there is to be some understanding of the implications on the quality of nursing relationships.

A profession can be defined as an occupational group which has a legally supported monopoly by a registration system. In the case of nurses this is the United Kingdom Central Council and the Nurses, Midwives and Health Visitors Act (1979). An occupational group which is able to control its own work, educational standards, entry into the profession, has professional autonomy over practice, and, perhaps most importantly, is only open to scrutiny by its peers, is a very powerful group. How this power is used is open to examination.

Johnson (1972) says that one of the main characteristics of a profession is the social distance and the unequal relationship between the professional and the clients, or, simply stated, that the more an occupational group seeks professional status the more it becomes socially distanced from its clients and recreates the inequality of society, in the professional–client relationship. Is the creation of an asymmetrical relationship what is really needed in nurse–patient relationships?

If nursing, as it would appear, is intent on pursuing the aim of professionalization, then there are inherent dangers. Much of nursing activity and nursing relationships should focus on a sense of 'being with' the patient, that is, holding and containing the patients' anxiety for them and being with them when they are at their most vulnerable. In professionalized relationships there is often an over-emphasis on 'doing to'. In these relationships, there is focus on technical expertise and practical procedures, which do not always take account of the patients' primitive anxiety.

The pursuit of professionalization creates high pressure on nurses and may well militate against them having a helpful, caring, nurturing relationship with patients.

## CREATING THE ENVIRONMENT TO USE SELF

For nurses to use their life experiences appropriately they need to give appropriate regard to the environment in which nursing activity takes place. Creating an appropriate environment is broader than simply ensuring an appropriate physical environment, it is also about creating the appropriate psychological environment. The way in which the psychological environment or space is created is important. The use of the word space in this context is deliberate. It acknowledges that personal psychological space to explore the internal feelings and anxieties that are created by being vulnerable and ill is as important as the technical and practical procedures.

The psychological space should lead the nurse to understand her position in the relationship. It should lead to the question: Why am I interacting in this way? Why did I say this in preference to that? What are my feelings in the relationship and what feelings belong to the patient? In order for the feelings and experiences of the nurses to be understandable they need to be placed within a framework which informs practice. There are numerous theoretical psychological models to inform practice and arguments will continue about which is the most appropriate. What is important is the ability to find a consistent model for oneself which is comfortable and allows understanding to develop.

Winnicott (1971 and 1981) had a clear framework for his work as a paediatrician. He was able to describe a psychological framework for his activity during a consultation with a mother and a child. Rather than just focus on the activity of the mother or the child he was able to describe a framework that recognized the relationship between himself as a paediatrician and the mother and child. In his work he created a psychological space with clearly defined boundaries that allowed the mother and child to experience their relationship and to work through the difficult and painful feelings that relationship engendered. This frame-work prevented Winnicott from intervening prematurely when it might have been inappropriate. It may have been that to intervene would have prevented the resolution of the feelings that both mother and child had in the relationship. Winnicott described the mother as physically holding the child and he (the doctor) psychologically holding the situation. Holding is a way of containing the anxiety created in relationships and provides a way of understanding the process.

Similarly, within nursing it is often the ward sister who psychologically holds the situation on the ward and often the staff nurse and health care assistant who physically hold (nurtures/nurses) the patient. Holding does not take place by accident—it is a combination of organizational structure, an internalization of theory and a recognition of the position of the self in the relationship. The actions of the nurse are informed by the process of holding, rather than being acted out in response to the patient's internal world and projections.

The actions of the nurse in the relationship should take into account the feelings of the patient as well as the feelings that are being felt but not acknowledged by the nurse. For example, Susan, a speech therapist, was a patient in the maternity unit following the birth of her first child. Sadly, the child was born with a cleft palate and a hare lip. Susan was clearly upset, but more distressed to find that nobody came to talk to her about it and she was moved to a side room. She eventually read her case notes, which were casually left at the bottom of her bed. Written in large red letters at the top of the page was 'mother is anxious +++'. Susan asked the staff nurse who looked after her why she had said that she was anxious about the cleft palate and hare lip when she had not discussed it with her. The staff nurse felt unable to explain her 'diagnosis' of anxiety but felt that because Susan was a speech therapist it must be impossible for her to bear the upset of her child's 'deformity'. She went on to say that she knew very little about the child's problems and prognosis. What is apparent is that the feelings that the staff nurse had about the child made her prejudge the situation. What would have been more appropriate would have been for her to acknowledge her own feelings about the baby and sit down with Susan to discuss hers. The staff nurse's own anxious feelings made Susan feel isolated and unsupported at a time of great stress. In this case the feelings in the nurse were clearly projected into the patient. It was not possible for the nurse to recognize which feelings belonged to her and which to the patient.

Sometimes the feelings that nurses have during interactions are positively helpful in helping the patient to understand their position and difficulties. Stephen was being seen by a community psychiatric nurse (CPN) on a weekly basis. He was 17 and living at home with his parents. He was referred because he was 'depressed and isolated'. He came along week after week, nothing apparently changing. The CPN found Stephen an increasingly irritating patient who made the nurse feel angry because he wouldn't change. Stephen seemed unable to generate any enthusiasm for anything. The CPN did not express his angry feelings in the sessions with the patient but discussed them in supervision. The supervisor and the nurse reflected on the meaning of the nurse's feelings and, more importantly, what they might mean in the context of the CPN's relationship with Stephen. At the next session the nurse said to Stephen that he felt angry at him at times in the sessions. Stephen, who usually had his head down, looked up, smiled and said 'My dad always says that'. Over the subsequent sessions Stephen was able to talk more about his relationship with his father. He said that as far as his father was concerned he was a failure and Stephen felt that nothing he could do or say would change that. Stephen described his intense feelings of anger at his father which previously had not been recognized or expressed. Stephen was slowly able to liberate himself from his painful feelings by exploring them in a safe, contained, structured environment. The recognition of the angry feelings in the nurse and the structured exploration of them allowed Stephen to express how he really felt. The recreation of his relationship with his father in the relationship with the CPN allowed Stephen to understand his anger about his father's disappointment, rather than simply acting it out as depression. As he became able to express his angry feeling directly to his father he no longer needed to feel depressed and isolated.

The appropriate recognition of the nurse's own feelings, the framework to understand those feelings and the ability to contain those feelings allowed a clear understanding of the difficulties that the patient was experiencing.

## TOWARDS SELF-AWARENESS

Becoming self-aware and being able to make good use of the self-awareness is not something which automatically occurs. Indeed several writers have reflected on the difficulty of teaching good communication skills in nursing practice (Faulkner *et al.*, 1983; Macleod Clarke, 1981; Hein, 1980). Nor is it appropriate to assume that self-awareness development is only important in basic training; there has to be consistent ongoing development of self-awareness throughout professional practice.

As nurses develop in their career they move from being in an anxious position about their relationships and ability, to a position of greater confidence. In this position of confidence they have a greater ability to tolerate the uncertainty and ambiguity of role. The greater experience and training nurses have, the less they feel they know. In nursing practice this is something that should be cultivated, rather than something to be afraid of.

It is not really realistic to expect that each individual nurse should bear the whole responsibility for their individual practice alone. The nurse is in a context and in a relationship with patients, colleagues and the organization she works for. It is important to think about the development of self-awareness in broader terms than focusing on the individual. It is perhaps helpful to consider three prerequisites which might need to met before self-awareness can develop fully.

First, organizational culture. It will not be possible to develop and use one's own feelings and experiences if the organizational culture in which one is operating is not receptive. If the idea that nurses' feelings should not be expressed is the dominant cultural norm, then any expression of emotion is going to be frowned on. The development of a culture which values the personal feelings, experiences and emotions of its nurses is not just the responsibility of one person. The whole organization must share the same cultural values and norms.

Secondly, a structured way of thinking about the relationship and the interaction. There are many frameworks and models for conceptualizing the meaning of the interaction and informing an appropriate response. Often these models, whether they be psychoanalytic, behavioural or cognitive, are seen as competing and different. Rather than using a multitude of models, it is often more sensible to use one that 'psychologically fits' the nurse. If a model or framework 'fits' it makes sense and is comfortable for the nurse. Smith (1979 and 1986) has outlined a useful framework to help student psychiatric nurses understand the process and content of their relationships. This framework has a wider application in all branches of nursing.

Finally, constant and consistent supervision. This is perhaps the most important element in enabling the use of self in the nursing relationship. The function of supervision is to enable and facilitate the process of the nursing relationship. It should not be seen as a hierarchical controlling relationship. However, the whole aim of this book is to discuss the notion of clinical supervision so it is inappropriate to discuss it further here.

## SUMMARY

This chapter has focused on the therapeutic use of self in the nursing relationship. The importance of acknowledging the context in which the relationship takes place has been discussed as well as the limitations, in terms of organizational structure, occupational stress and the pursuit of professionalization of nursing. The broad way in which the environmental conditions have to be correct and created to use self are discussed. Finally, there is a brief description of the prerequisites for making appropriate use of self in the nurse–patient relationship.

## REFERENCES

Best, G. (1987) *The Future of NHS General Management: Where Next?*, Kings Fund College.

Davis, M. and Wallbridge, D. (1981) *Boundary and Space; an Introduction to the Work of D. W. Winnicott*, Karmac.

DHSS (1983) *Health Care and its Costs*, HMSO, London.

Doyle, L. (1979) *The Political Economy of Health*, Pluto Press, London.

Faulkner, A., Bridge, W., Macleod Clarke, J. and Williams, A. (1983) *Teaching Communication Skills in Nursing*, Paper given at RCN Research Conference at Brighton in 1983.

Gamble, A. M. and Walkland, S. A. (1984) *The British Party System and Economic Policy 1945–1983*, Clarendon Press, London.

Gowler, D. and Parry, G. (1983) Career Stresses on Psychological Therapists, in *Psychology and Psychotherapy, Current Trends and Issues* (Ed. D. Pilgrim), Routledge and Kegan Paul, London.

Hein, E. C. (1980) *Communication in Nursing Practice*, Little Brown, Boston.

Illich, I. (1977) *Limits to Medicine, Medical Nemesis: The Expropriation of Health*, Penguin, London.

Johnson, T. J. (1972) *Professions and Power*, Macmillan, London.

Klein, R. (1985) Health Policy 1979–1983: The Retreat from Ideology?, in *Implementing Government Policy Initiatives* (Ed. P. M. Jackson), RIPA, London.

Macleod Clarke, J. (1981) Communication in nursing, *Nursing Times*, **77**(1), 12–18.

Maslach, C. (1976) Burned out, *Human Behaviour*, **5**, 16–22.

Maslach, C. and Jackson, S. E. (1981) Measurement of experienced burnout, *Journal of Occupational Behaviour*, **2**, 99–113.

Menzies, I. E. P. (1959) The functioning of social systems as a defence against anxiety: a report on a study of the nursing service of a general hospital, *Human Relations*, **13**, 95–121.

Menzies Lyth, I. E. P. (1988) *Containing Anxiety in Institutions, Selected Essays*, Free Association Books, London.

Navarro, V. (1976) *Medicine under Capitalism*, Prodist, New York.

Smith, L. (1979) Communication skills, *Nursing Times*, **75**(22), 926–9.

Smith, L. (1986) Talking it out, *Nursing Times*, **82**(13), 38–43.

Wilding, P. (1982) *Professional Power and Social Welfare*, Routledge and Kegan Paul, London.

Winnicott, D. W. (1971) *Therapeutic Consultations in Child Psychiatry*, Hogarth Press, London.

# CHAPTER FOUR

# Providing support and reducing stress: a review of the literature

*Katie Booth*

## INTRODUCTION

Clinical supervision clearly has a part to play in the provision of support to nurses and may provide a vehicle for stress reduction. There is some evidence that clinical supervision has been attempted through group work and has been variously reported on. The results are often contradictory and it is clear that there is much work to be done in evaluating the usefulness of support and stress reduction. What follows is a review of some of the debate.

The evidence that social support is useful in explaining some individual differences of vulnerability to adverse circumstances has led to interest in its effects in occupational settings. For example, Marcellisen (1988) uses four aspects of social support – emotional support, appraisal support, affirmative feedback and information support – in his study of social support and work. The basic premise of his study was that strong social support could be expected to protect against job stressors. This study has many of the features which interest workers in the field of health care. There has been an assumption that work will be stressful and that certain aspects of social support might be thought to protect the vulnerable in a work setting. Marcellisen's findings were not clear cut. Results suggested that people at the top and the bottom of the hierarchy felt they received least social support, that only with the lower occupational groups did social support seem to protect against stressors, that support from co-workers did not seem to be as effective as from supervisors and that, indeed, colleague relationships may deteriorate when the individual experiences occupational strains.

The four-strand approach to social support is proposed by House 1981. His concept refers to the flow of one or more elements between people: emotional concern, instrumental aid, information and appraisal.

## SUPPORT AND HEALTH CARE WORKERS

It is the potential for social support to protect workers from pressure which concerns writers from the health care professions where occupational stress is thought to be very common. Many studies have demonstrated that carers feel under pressure (Cooper, 1988; MacKay, 1988) and much of this work concerns nurses (Wolfgang, 1988). Hingley and Harris (1986) make the point that, until very recently, the nursing profession has tended to neglect the idea of professional support and consider occupational pressures as the problem of the individual nurse. Their study of senior nurses showed a lack of support and uncovered much distress. For instance, of the sample of charge nurses and above, 85% considered that they were overloaded by pressure of work and there was a widespread perception of being short of the staff needed to perform a worthwhile job. Of the respondents, 60% found involvement with life and death situations upsetting. Over half felt that the only feedback they received was negative, that they were only told about those aspects of their performance that were judged to be unsatisfactory. Professional support from superiors was lacking and was cited as a major source of distress. Baider and Porath (1981) spoke of uncovering a climate of fear amongst all grades in a cancer ward and Tschudin (1985) suggests that recent changes in the philosophy of care have made nurses feel insecure and personally guilty where organizations do not offer professional guidance.

Burnout has been defined as a syndrome of emotional exhaustion, depersonalization and a reduced sense of personal accomplishment, which can occur among individuals who work with people in some capacity (Maslach and Jackson, 1986). Leiter and Maslach (1988) examined the interpersonal relationships between nurses in a small general hospital. Three aspects of the interpersonal environment were related to the three concepts of burnout. Pleasant supervisor and co-worker contact were related to positive employee feelings, such as personal accomplishment and commitment; negative contact, especially from the supervisor, was related to burnout. Hare, Pratt and Andrews (1988) suggest that low social support at work enhances vulnerability to burnout and Yasko (1983) reports a lack of perceived psychological support at work as being a predicting factor.

Browner (1987) showed carers with supportive work-based social relationships having a more positive profile on the Cornell Medical Index. Norbeck (1985) found social support to be negatively related to perceived job stress in critical care nursing but that social support did not seem to protect the worker from the psychological symptoms thought to result from perceived job stress (buffering). This is interesting in the light of the study by Winnubst *et al.* (1982), who from a large sample of Dutch industrial organizations produced evidence that not only was social support from the supervisor and co-workers negatively related to job stressors, psychological and behavioural strains and with several health problems, but also that there were lower co-relations to support the buffering of the impact of some work-related stressor (psychological and behavioural), but not health strains. The evidence in this large study (1246 employees) of the buffering effects of social support against job stressors is reported as disappointing.

In a hospice study (Smith, 1985), nurses were asked about their perceptions of support. The most frequent attribute of support was non-judgemental listening, the second was encouragement, and assistance (physical help) came third. Nurses expressed a clear need for support with aspects of caring for dying patients and their relatives. They expected and received this help from each other. Further, there is some evidence that these relationships may influence the planning and delivery of care (Peterson, 1988).

## NEED FOR ACTION

Many writers consider that these felt pressures and deficits in support constitute a serious problem—one which has grave implications for nurses and their work—and suggestions are made for individual, interpersonal and organizational action to support nurses and other health care workers in order to protect them (Bolle, 1988; Cox, 1988; Crawley, 1988; Sparkes, 1989; Hingley and Cooper, 1986).

However, at present there seems to be a lack of information which managers could use to justify these initiatives. A review by Owen (1990) for the National Association of Staff Support Within the Health Care Services, an organization which has been recently formed to promote staff support, discusses the experience of both the United States and this country. She says: 'there is little evidence on the cost effectiveness of support systems although anecdotal accounts indicate strong relationships with staff and patient turnover also staff morale, absenteeism and general standards of patient care'. She also points out that costs and resourcing staff support work are seldom considered.

## THE NATURE OF THE WORK

There is a commonly held assumption that it is the unique nature of caring work per se which gives rise to these difficulties, but this is questionable. For instance, high technology care, with its very sick patients, complex machinery and ethical dilemmas, is much quoted as having adverse effects upon the nurse and her ability to care (Bailey *et al.*, 1980; Biley, 1989; Wilson-Barnett, 1984). However, it has been shown by Nichols (1981) that intensive care units need not be felt as distressing by nurses. Items such as patient care and interpersonal relationships in intensive care units are regarded as being the most potentially rewarding as well as the most potentially disturbing aspect of the work. In some units there were very high levels of job satisfaction and morale, but the reverse was true in other units. Conclusions from this study were that the distress often reported may be more of a comment on aspects of the individual situation, such as style of leadership, than on the specialty of nursing. The complexity of these situations is supported by a small study of hospice nursing (Barstow, 1980). Here, nurses were unhappy about specific aspects of their work, such as not being able to control patients' symptoms and difficult work schedules, but when their anxiety states were measured (Spielberger) much lower scores were found than the author had been led to believe from the literature. That there may be some individual as well as situational differences is demonstrated by two further studies. Shinn *et al.* (1984) reported a difference between men and women in the caring services, and they suggested that the female carers had more access to social support thereby producing differing responses to stress, but when Parkes (1986) looked at individual differences between student nurses and at the coping styles they employed, the conclusion was that the nature of the work environment accounted for the largest proportion of variance in the coping styles reported. It is clear that much work remains to be done in this area before more positive correlations can be seen.

## INITIATIVES TO HELP

Various group settings have been described where the aim has been to enhance professional achievement. For instance Richman and Rosenfield (1987) suggest that:

> groupwork matches individual needs and resources to improve the functioning of the person within her or his environment, and groupwork provides mutual aid wherein each member mutually supports the achievement of group and person goals.

There are others who take a very similar view. Diminno and Thompson (1980) set up a group to help with professional and personal issues and increase self-awareness. The members liked it and felt the approach used was relevant. Gaumont and Dwarak (1980), discussing support for nurses in an oncology unit, reported early problems in that group members needed to be 'reminded' of the sessions (taking 30 min to gather staff together, many being unable to attend, etc.). The group improved over time.

At evaluation, positive feelings were reported about the group, e.g. 'tremendous sense of relief to learn that other nurses had similar feelings'. Scully (1981) describes a group set up to provide personal support to nurses, and reports that 'nurses began to help each other and patient care improved'.

However, when evaluations of this type of activity contain more structured methods of measurement, the benefits become less clear. Silberfarb and Levine (1980) describe group support for oncology nurses. Outcome measures were made using a semantic differential list focused on job-related concepts. The nurses, who were all volunteers, were reported to be appreciative of the group experience, but unfortunately their attitudes to job-related concepts changed in a negative direction. The control group of nurses who did not volunteer to attend the groups showed less negative changes. On the other hand, Razavi *et al.* (1988) report changes in the desired attitudinal direction after training sessions with carers of the terminally ill, those with the most negative attitudes showing most change.

With regard to academic pressures, Mitchell *et al.* (1983) were unable to demonstrate measurable effects on the academic performance of medical students who had attended support groups. Neither were any effects seen in terms of measures of anxiety (Speilberger) or depression (Beck).

A managerial measure sometimes used in this type of work is sickness absence and Milne, Walker and Bamford (1987), in an admittedly very small study (seven health visitors), found no change after support sessions.

## REDUCING STRESS

Stress reduction is often seen as a goal for professional support and programmes of support are often evaluated by examining measures of stress. For example, Grey Toft (1980) set up initiatives aimed at the 'Facilitation of staff support programmes, whereby health care professionals are assisted to cope more effectively with the stress of the hospital environment'. There were measurements of stress, the self-reported nursing stress scale and managerial measures (a job satisfaction sub-scale of a Job Description Index). Hospice staff (17 in all) participated in the group sessions, and the study, which had a controlled design, reported lower stress measures and higher job satisfaction after work in the groups. Positive managerial results are reported in a study in which autogenic regulation training was provided for nurses in training (Bailey, 1984). In this study, nurses in the training group had fewer days away from work than a control group.

There are often accounts by enthusiastic writers who report stress reduction and professional benefits to the nurse from group attendance. The professional benefits included feelings of mutual support, better work performance and job satisfaction. These tend to be based on members' comments, for example, Nicholas (1987), Appleby (1987) or Skinner (1980).

Richman and Rosenfield (1987) found that groups were not always successful in meeting their stress reduction aims. When outcomes were measured, it seemed that involvement in a group per se did not affect reported stress, neither did the amount of external support available to each member, whereas the type of group attended did. On the basis of questionnaires returned from 54% of the sample (151 subjects), self-reported stress levels improved in groups which helped the hospice workers by being challenging in terms of both technical and emotional issues; there was sharing of social reality but not non-judgemental listening support.

On the basis of this work, Richman (1988) has proposed a model for groups to 'buffer stress' and therefore reduce burnout. He proposes technical challenge, emotional challenge, shared social reality and non-judgemental listening to be encouraged outside the work-related social group.

Other authors report negative results in studies aimed at the alleviation of distress, e.g. McClam (1980), and Mullins and Merriam (1983) who examined the effects of programmes to address death anxiety. In a support group popular with its members, which was intended to help hospice staff, Larson (1986) was unable to demonstrate that burnout scores were significantly affected by support group attendance.

## ACCEPTABILITY

There is some evidence that nurses do not necessarily like groups, nor are prepared to attend them. For example Appleby (1987) reported that a quarter of members (three out of the 12) found that the groups were unhelpful or stopped attending. It also seems likely that the idea of professional support in groups is not universally accepted by the nurses. Silberfarb and Levine found that 17 out of 29 oncology nurses were not prepared to attend the groups, and used them as controls. Booth and Faulkner (1986) found nurses reluctant to attend support sessions and very wary of their colleagues, whilst Diminno and Thompson (1980) show that only one-third of nurses eligible volunteered for a support group.

Galinsky and Schlopler (1977) (social workers) warn that 'groups may be dangerous' and they write from their own experiences of members who felt group work had been to their disadvantage, suggesting that a 16% 'casualty' rate is to be expected. Galinsky describes ways in which group leaders can minimize such casualties, for instance, screening members and leaders, provision of both external support and evaluation of group functioning. Other authors share this concern. There is some consensus that in order to be as safe as possible such groups should take account of nurses' likely needs for confidentiality. Also considered important are a mix of colleagues with whom they feel comfortable, and the fostering of a safe trusting atmosphere facilitated by someone outside the organizational hierarchy (Gaumont and Dwarak, 1989; Epting, 1981; Corey and Corey, 1977; Booth and Faulkner, 1986).

## DISCUSSION

On the whole support for nurses seems to be provided in order to prevent high turnover and burnout, and to increase job satisfaction. Conclusions about the professional support for health care workers are rather difficult to draw and this may be partly because many of the experimental studies described have used very small samples.

A more serious problem is that definitions and operationalizations of the concepts of professional support, social support and stress vary widely and are not always clearly made. In addition, groups set up for stress reduction sometimes use indirect managerial outcomes, such as sickness rates, whilst on the other hand some which aim to promote professional support use stress measures as outcomes.

It is also not clear if the type of help currently on offer is necessary or acceptable to all nurses, or if there are alternative ways of promoting and measuring staff well-being. In terms of patient care, there still seems to be a question about professional support. Is it related to the ability or willingness to engage in certain aspects of meeting patients' needs, for example their emotional needs?

## SUMMARY OF THE LITERATURE

1. There does seem a great deal of reported distress and unhappiness amongst nurses.
2. Groups and other initiatives do not always distinguish between professional support and relief of distress.
3. Deliberate attempts to alleviate distress may meet with approval from the health workers concerned, but it is more difficult to show benefit in terms of standard psychological or managerial measures. An

explanation here could be that the measures used may not always have been suitable to the type of intervention, the numbers may have been inadequate and the design of the help offered may be a major factor, i.e. a non-directive approach may be less helpful.

In a similar way professional support groups aimed at discussion and help with work-related issues may show positive results, but mainly when the evaluation uses a non-standard measure.

4. Group work may not suit everyone, and should be led by trained facilitators, preferably non-members of the organizational hierarchy. Not all nurses will attend deliberate help sessions when they are given a choice.

5. Not all nurses report distress; when they do it seems to be that the individual setting is more important than the specialty. The perceived managerial and interpersonal environment seems to be important in terms of happiness at work.

6. The question of professional support and clinical activity needs further exploration.

## REFERENCES

Appleby, F. M. (1987) Professional support and the role of support groups, *Health Visitor*, **60**, 77–78.

Baider, L. and Porath, S. (1981) Uncovering fear: group experience of nurses in a cancer ward, *International Journal of Nursing Studies*, **18**, 47–52.

Bailey, J. T., Steffen, S. M. and Grout, J. W. (1980) The stress audit: Identifying the stresses of ICU nursing, *Journal of Nurse Education*, **19**, 15–26.

Bailey, R. D. (1984) Autogenic regulation training and sickness absence amongst student nurses in general training, *Journal of Advanced Nursing*, **9**, 581–587.

Barstow, J. (1980) Stress variance in hospice nursing, *Nursing Outlook*, December, 751–754.

Biley, F. C. (1989) Stress in high dependency units, *Intensive Care Nursing*, **5**, 134–141.

Bolle, J. L. (1988) Supporting the deliverers of care, *Nursing Clinics of North America*, **23**(4), 843–850.

Booth, K. and Faulkner, A. (1986) Problems encountered in setting up support groups in nursing, *Nurse Education Today*, **6**, 244–251.

Browner, C. H. (1987) Job stress and health: The role of social support at work, *Research in Nursing and Health*, **10**, 93–100.

Cooper, C. (1988) *Stress Mental Health and Job Satisfaction*, Health Services Management Research 1.1.

Corey, G. and Corey, M. S. (1977) *Groups Process and Practice*, Brooks/Cole Montery, California.

Cox, C. (1988) Practical aspects of stress management, *British Journal of Occupational Therapy*, **51**(2), 44–47.

Crawley, P. (1988) Giving good counsel, *Nursing Standard*, 25 June.

Diminno, M. and Thompson, E. (1980) An interactional support group for graduate nursing students, *Journal of Nursing Education*, **19**(3), 16–22.

Epting, S. P. (1981) Coping with stress through peer support, *Topics in Clinical Nursing*, **4**, 47–49.

Galinsky, M. J. and Schlopler, J. H. (1988) Warning: Groups may be dangerous, *Social Work*, **22**, 89–94.

Gaumont, B. and Dwarak, M. H. (1980) Group work with nurses, *Health and Social Work*, **5**(3), 76–77.

Hare, J., Pratt, C. C. and Andrews, D. (1988) Predictors of burnout in professional and para-professional nurses, *International Journal of Nursing Studies*, **25**(2), 105–115.

Hingley, P. and Cooper, C. L. (1986) *Stress and the Nurse Manager*, J. Wiley & Sons, Chichester.

Hingley, P. and Harris, P. (1986) Burnout at senior level, *Nursing Times*, **82**(31), 28–29, **82**(32), 52–53.

House, J. S. (1981) *Barriers to Work Stress 1 Social Support in Behavioral Medicine*, Work Stress and Health (Eds. Gentry *et al.*), Martinus, Dordrecht.

Larson, D. G. (1986) Developing effective hospice staff support groups, *Hospice Journal*, **2**(2), 41–55.

Leiter, M. P. and Maslach, C. (1988) The impact of interpersonal environment on burnout and organizational commitment, *Journal of Organizational Behaviour*, **9**(4), 297–308.

MacKay, L. (1988) Career women, *Nursing Times*, **84**(10), 42–43, (10), 33–34.

Marcelissen, F. H. G., Winnubst, J. A. M., Buunk, B. and De Wolff, C. J. (1988) Social support and occupational stress: A causal analysis, *Social Science and Medicine*, **26**(3), 365–373.

Maslach, C. and Jackson, S. E. (1986) *Maslach Burnout Inventory Manual*, 2nd edn, Consulting Psychologists Press, Plato Alto CA.

McClam, T. (1980) Death anxiety before and after death education: negative results, *Psychological Reports*, **46**, 513–514.

Milne, D., Walker, L. and Bamford, S. (1987) Professional coping, *Health Visitor*, **6**, 49–50.

Mitchell, R. E., Matthews, J. R., Grundy, T. G. and Lupo, J. L. (1983) The question of stress among first year medical students, *Journal of Medical Education*, **58**, 367–372.

Mullins, L. C. and Merriam, S. (1983) The effects of short term death training programmes on nursing home staff, *Death Education*, **7**, 352–368.

Nicholas, K. A., Springford, V. and Serle, J. (1981) An investigation into distress and discontent in various types of nursing, *Journal of Advanced Nursing*, **6**, 311–318.

Nicholas, V. B. (1987) Stress management programme counters emotional burnout, *Provider*, **13**(3), 42–44.

Norbeck, J. S. (1985) Types and sources of social support for managing job stress in critical care nursing, *Nursing Research*, **30**, 225–230.

Owen, G. (1990) *Coping with Stress: Support Networks for Professional Carers*, Artemis Trust.

Parkes, K. R. (1986) Coping in stressful episodes: The role of individual difference, environmental factors and situational characteristics, *Journal of Personality and Social Psychology*, **51**, 1277–1292.

Peterson, M. (1988) The norms and values held by three groups of nurses concerning psychosocial nursing practice, *International Journal of Nursing Studies*, **25**(2), 85–103.

Razavi, D., Delvaux, N., Farvacques, C. and Robaye, E. (1988) Immediate effectiveness of brief psychological training for health professionals dealing with terminally ill cancer patients, *Social Science and Medicine*, **27**(4), 369–375.

Richman, J. M. (1988) Social support groups, *Journal of Nursing Administration*, **18**(2), 3, 19.

Richman, J. M. and Rosenfield, L. B. (1987) Stress reduction in hospice workers: A support group model, *Hospice Journal*, **3**(2/3), 205–221.

Scully, R. (1981) Staff support groups, *Journal of Nursing Administration*, **11**(3), 48–51.

Shinn, M., Rosario, M., Morch, H. and Chestnut, D. E. (1984) Coping with job stress and burnout in the human services, *Journal of Personality and Social Psychology*, **46**, 4, 863–876.

Silberfarb, P. M. and Levine, P. M. (1980) Psychosocial aspects of neoplastic disease: Group support for the oncology nurse, *General Hospital Psychiatry*, **3**, 192–197.

Skinner, K. (1980) Support groups for ICU nurses, *Nursing Outlook*, May, 296–299.

Smith, S. P. (1985) Hospice: A supportive working environment for nurses, *Journal of Palliative Care*, **1**(1), 16–23.

Sparkes, T. F. (1989) Coping with the psychological stresses of oncology care, *Journal of Psychological Oncology*, **6**(1/2), 165–179.

Tschudin, V. (1985) Too much pressure, *Nursing Times*, **81**(37), 30–31, **81**(38), 45–46.

Wilson-Barnett, J. (1984) Coping with stress, *Nursing Mirror*, **158**(14), s. 16.

Winnubst, J. A. M., Marcelissen, F. H. G. and Kleber, R. J. (1982) Effects of social support in the stressor–strain relationship: A Dutch sample, *Social Science and Medicine*, **16**, 475–482.

Wolfgang, A. P. (1988) Job stress in the health professions, *Behavioral Medicine*, **14**(1), 43–47.

Yasko, J. M. (1983) Variables which predict burnout experienced by oncology clinical nurse specialists, *Cancer Nursing*, April, 109–116.

# PART TWO

# Professional and Practice Perspectives

## INTRODUCTION

This section of the book is a presentation by various subject specialists to clinical supervision in their clinical areas. The contributors have not followed a common format; indeed their definitions are very far apart on some occasions but at other times almost identical. This is intentional, and there are no attempts to squeeze out a common definition which suits all areas. Rather, as the reader will see, this part of the book attempts to highlight developments which others may find useful. Not surprisingly the different clinical areas have their own vocabulary and have developed ideas which best serve themselves. It is for the reader to draw from the different chapters those ideas which they find helpful and make of them what they will in their own clinical areas. What follows in the next nine chapters is a distillation of various ideas on clinical supervision in nursing, and a brief look at some of the ideas presented serves to underwrite their general usefulness.

Psychiatric nursing has a particular interest in interpersonal matters of this sort and Philip Barker draws our attention to the power relationships which can be both profitable but at the same time dangerous as he reminds us that 'the more useful we are to people the more useless they can become'. More profitably he shows that supervision can be a time to gain an awareness of choices. Paediatric nursing is presented by Barbara Elliot as a service in which non-nurses can have a part to play in the supervision of children at play. Indeed parents are shown to be critical in the supervision of nurses caring for their children.

Partnership and clinical supervision takes on a new meaning where parents and their children can be more knowledgeable about their condition than their carers. Penny Curtis presents the supervision of midwives as a case study of some of the problems of asserting control over more independent practice, highlighting the complex social relationships which can affect practice, autonomy and supervision. She shows through reported observations how subtle forces play in what are at first sight unremarkable everyday events.

Jane Merchant explains how general nursing has been influenced by the ways that nursing work is organized and the effects that primary nursing and team nursing have had on clinical supervision. She highlights the dilemmas of frequently changing personnel and the inherent 'risks' of being a delegator.

Mental handicap nursing is shown by Peggy Cooke to have considerable experience in multi-disciplinary working and that this in itself provides a challenge as the work of nurses has a more public scrutiny. Case conferencing and the use of video equipment are seen to have value in promoting good practice.

Sheila Twinn has studied the work of health visitors and presents her work on the preparation for practice which is undertaken by health visitor students. She discusses how these students (often already well experienced general nurses) need a protected environment with careful supervision to prepare them for their new experiences. She also puts forward some explanation of the difficulty of acting as a role model, teacher and assessor.

Robert Nettleton presents research work he has conducted with health visitors and their duties relating to child protection. In this most difficult and sensitive area he explores the ways in which health visitors deal with the uncertainty of the case work presented to them. Often ill-defined and anxiety provoking, this is an area of case work which demands the highest skill and yet presents no clear answers. Health visitors will be dealing with other professionals whom they must trust, colleagues they need to turn to for support and managers with whom they must share matters which are difficult to express.

Marion Balcombe introduces occupational health nursing and suggests that there are inherent problems with working independently, often as a lone worker. She highlights the difficulty of providing clinical supervision and suggests that there is some stress in constantly guarding against errors of judgement without the benefit of peer support.

Brian Pateman shows that, like health visiting, district nursing has a considerable tradition of student supervision and the concept of gradually exposing students to more responsible and autonomous practice. He presents the findings from a small local survey which demonstrates the variety of ways that district nursing is carrying out clinical supervision with its qualified and more experienced staff.

The final chapter in this part of the book comes from community psychiatric nursing. Peter Wilkin discusses the increasing attention that community psychiatric nurses are giving to mentorship and clinical supervision as they have had to accommodate moving from hospital-based team nursing to independent practice, with sometimes only limited preparation. It is possible to take something from all these chapters and place it in any nursing setting: the specialty is unimportant, the lessons are universal.

# CHAPTER FIVE

# Psychiatric nursing

## *Phil Barker*

While she was away I thought she must be a very new nurse: she had not yet become inhuman, but was trying to learn the trick. (Welch, 1983)

## ARMING OURSELVES

People who think they know what is best for others should not be taken too seriously. Indeed, as some have suggested such people may even be dangerous (Rowe, 1989). Any consideration of psychiatric nursing, its practice and its value must, therefore, accommodate the unknown as a balance for what little knowledge we do possess.

It is commonly accepted that quality psychiatric nursing involves the 'therapeutic use of self'. Some North American nurses have long argued that this activity, or rather its expression through interpersonal relationships, is the very basis of psychiatric nursing (Peplau, 1986). Travelbee (1971) has noted, for example, that nursing 'is an interpersonal process because it is always concerned with people either directly or indirectly'. This principle is clearly relevant, however, to just about every other caring group. Butterworth (1987) has declared the patent need for British psychiatric nurses to demonstrate expertise in interpersonal relationships and therapeutic use of self, suggesting that the fine detail of such activity might in some way distinguish the ideology of psychiatric nursing. The long pedigree of interpersonal relationship building skills and theory possessed by North American nurses is beyond challenge (Schwartz and Shockley, 1956). It is not yet clear, however, whether British nurses' current interest in the same territory represents an equivalent ideology, science of ideas, or reflection of a consistent theoretical rationale

(Altschul, 1972). It can be accepted as a canon of faith that the nurse's manipulation of her/himself, during contact with the person who is the patient, characterizes psychiatric nursing practice. It is less easy to believe, however, that nurses, or the people in their care, always understand what exactly is taking place.

The significance of what exactly is meant by 'self' and therefore its therapeutic use is critical to the area of supervision in psychiatric nursing. It is an unsafe assumption that any psychiatric nurse possesses only one 'self' which is manipulated to positive effect with a wide range of people in care across a range of situations.

I suspect that nurses often use 'themselves' as a subtle controlling, manipulative force, in an effort to change the people in their care, somehow 'for the better'. This is not only characteristic of nurses, but all carers, professional or lay, who are inclined to feel guilty when 'not doing enough'. The therapeutic use of self can be benign and kindly, or it can be openly challenging and confrontational. Some would argue that the attempt to make people conform, whether subtle or gross, is an outstanding characteristic of all psychotherapies (Masson, 1989), hence the current concern for the emotional security of all who might be offered help which involves the professional's 'therapeutic use of self'.

## DISARMING

Supervision in psychiatric nursing has two main aims: to protect people in care from nurses and to protect nurses from themselves. In dealing with the protection of people in care I do not wish to address issues involving the overt, intentional, abuse of people in care, although I am aware that examples of malpractice continue to be reported. Rather, I wish to focus on situations where people in care receive unnecessary or over-zealous direction from nurses who believe that they know what is 'best'. Given my belief that nurses should be involved in 'empowering' people in care, this might be termed a problem of benign paternalism. Psychiatric medicine, like its mainstream equivalent, involves the treatment of people with mental disorder, with or without their consent. Psychiatric nursing may manipulate aspects of the person's 'illness' as part of care, but is not concerned directly with treatment. Nursing manipulates the person's relationship with illness.

## THE HELPING RELATIONSHIP

A distinction needs to be made here between the related concepts of 'helpfulness' and 'helping'. Nurses are portrayed, traditionally, as professionals who try to be helpful. Invariably this means that they intervene on behalf of the person in care. Nurses who guide a person away from danger in the direction of safety are, quite reasonably, seen to be helpful. Preventing a person from harming himself, or others, is a helpful action. Calming people who are anxious and frightened, raising the spirits of those who are in despair, can all be seen as helpful. Such actions, however, have little to do with the promotion of growth and development. Indeed, dependency in its various forms can be traced directly to the helpful actions of nurses and others. Clearly, nurses need to 'be helpful' in their everyday work with people in care. Such helpful actions are part and parcel of any social system in which interdependence is the rule and genuine independence is rare. Helpfulness is the support system which characterizes all social units. It is, therefore, an integral part of nursing. In my view it is not the most important part of nursing. We should not lose sight of the fact, however, that the more useful we are, the more useless the person might become.

Helping is about arranging ways of promoting growth and development. Often, such actions begin with something akin to 'being helpful', but thereafter the controlling emphasis moves gradually from the nurse to the person in care. People can experience sudden waves of emotion which precipitate aggressive acts, panic–flight–fright behaviour, or may 'paralyse' them. Highlighting the significant events or the person's thoughts or beliefs about the situation may 'be helpful' in clarifying the experience for the person. The nurse may be able to use such information as a basis for developing some alternative way of responding to, or dealing with, such situations. This may also be seen as 'helpful'. The challenge for the nurse lies in being able to transfer her part in this interpretation, clarification, resolution to the person in care. If she fails to do this the person will become dependent upon her as a means of resolving her emotional problems.

## THE MEANING OF LIFE

The psychological or psychiatric problems discussed above represent, in my view, problems of living. Although we are emphasizing here 'mental' problems, the difficulties experienced by people with a long-term physical illness or disability would be similar. Living with an amputation, unstable diabetes or memory defect following head injury, creates enormous problems of everyday living. Nurses, and other health-care professionals, are often tempted to express understanding of the disability: 'we know how you feel'. Helping a person identify, confront, overcome or otherwise manage a life problem requires our awareness of what such a problem might mean for us. The care of older people, which has at least in recent years been characterized by appalling standards of care, serves

as a good example of the problem we face in pursuing true understanding
of the person's problems of living.

Although it would be convenient for us to believe that some older
people experience a 'second childhood', this is hardly correct. From
middle age onwards our mastery of our bodies, our emotions and of
reality is reversed. Life is, for all of us, an onward march to the grave:
there is no going back, except in our imagination. Older people can be,
indeed often are, treated like children, when their faculties begin to fail
them. Such care fails to acknowledge what the experience of ageing and
diminishing capability might mean to the older person. We need to
consider whether or not such 'care' is a reflection of our own inadequacy
in dealing with the inevitability of decay and death.

Understanding, which is at the heart of all care, may be hard to come
by, especially where the young and beautiful are forced to confront the
transitory nature of their suppleness and good looks.

Physical empathy involves our 'understanding' of the vulnerability
which we share with the afflicted person in our care. Where physical
pathology is concerned we often console ourselves with the notion that
our chance of being similarly affected is either remote or that an effective
remedy would be available. Young people probably still pretend, as my
own generation did, that they hope they'll die before they get old.

Psychological empathy is more intimidating. It involves our understanding of the emotional experience of the person. Here too, the nurse
identifies strongly with the person, who unwittingly holds up a mirror to
his carer. Often the reflection is too hard too bear; the background
awareness that there is no panacea for emotional suffering, that
psychological distress often simply has to run its course, can be borne
easily only by the stoical or the wise. The easiest options are to deny the
experience in ourselves, or to diminish the importance of the experience
for the person. Given the psychological threat involved in empathic
relationships it is little wonder that people in care often feel that few
really understand them. When the nurse says 'I know how you feel' she
may merely be mouthing a worthless cliché or dealing with a mere
hypothesis.

'This is how I would feel if I were in your shoes: thankfully I'm not!'
This is a fragile kind of understanding. To be empathic we need to focus
all our attention on the person's description of his experience. Ironically,
we might appear to possess more understanding if we professed it less.
Goffman (1968) described the manipulation of the patient [sic] as
'degradation therapy' whereby he was obliged to take on the staff's
version of himself as a necessary condition of treatment. Manipulation is
also possible in a more benign form whenever carers exercise a belief that
they know 'what is happening within the person'. Although some people

in care may find it difficult to describe their experiences, carers need to question what is to be gained by advocating that they accept our construction of their reality. Holding back from making such interpretations can be immensely difficult, especially where nurses assume that such interpretations are at the very heart of psychiatric practice. Helping nurses to consider how they view and respond to the person's experience is one of the supervisor's tasks.

The special characteristic of psychiatric nursing involves the nurse's 'use of self' in the medium of the helping process. Although, as noted earlier, psychiatric nurses can also provide 'helpful', short-term interventions, the nature of such 'helpful' actions and the process by which they can be developed (preceptorship) does not differ significantly from other branches of nursing. 'Learning the ropes' involves the supervisor asking the question 'How can I help you meet this standard?'. The truly special demands of psychiatric nursing require the supervisor to ask a much more fundamental question: 'What is it that you need to do?' (Keith-Lucas, 1972). From this base grows a range of questions which increase in complexity the simpler they become: 'Are you aware of the alternatives? How do you know you can do that? What do you think will happen? How will you decide? What do you need me for?' The supervisor is not in a position of determining what needs to be done, although this may be very clear in her own mind. Rather, she is concerned to establish whether or not the novice is clear about her objectives and, more importantly, is willing to do what needs to be done. Given the emphasis upon interpersonal relationships, psychiatric nursing is a potential emotional minefield. Supervision is largely about helping the nurse to know what are her choices and to decide whether or not she is ready to take them.

## THE FOCUS ON THE PERSON

The focus on the person in care, the process of caring for him, and the acknowledgement of the nurse's needs, are intertwined. For the purpose of clarifying each of these I shall deal with them separately. Issues concerning the nurse's relationship with the person begin with their first meeting and end, literally, when last they meet. This relationship is, therefore, the ground upon which the care plan is laid, running the very length of their encounter. The stages involved in identifying and clarifying the person's needs, trying to meet them and evaluating their outcome, can be distinguished as units of the care plan. This distinction is, however, artificial since needs are more likely to be stated, re-stated and adapted throughout the helping encounter, as are the means of helping deployed by the nurse. Psychiatric nursing, if it is to be anything, should be an organic process. The nurse's helping should be integrated fully with the needs and nature of the person in care, in the same way as a plant co-exists with the soil from which it gains its sustenance and support. The supervisor needs to be aware of the organic nature of the care process under review: the supervisory process needs to be similarly reflexive and diffuse.

Despite this diffuse nature there clearly exists a need for structure upon which to base the supervisory process. In reality, the nurse's relationship with the person in care will ebb and flow, from involvement in discrete goal-orientated activities to contemplation and reflection. The nurse's experience of caring will change in a similar fashion: at times she will be more aware of herself than of the person; at others the 'activity' will override them both. It may be helpful to begin by examining these different relationships.

## The Relationships

Given the assumed interpersonal basis of psychiatric nursing, attention needs to be paid to the interaction of nurse and 'patient'. The founding father of the 'interpersonal school' of psychiatry, Harry Stack Sullivan, saw all psychiatry as:

> the study of processes that involve or go on between people. The field of interpersonal relations, under any and all circumstances in which these relations exist . . . a personality can never be isolated from the complex of interpersonal relations in which the person lives and has his being. (Sullivan, 1947, p. 4)

It may be most expedient to look at the relationship from the nurse's viewpoint, since she is the 'reporter'. The supervisor should not lose sight of the fact that the relationship is reciprocal, and the nurse may need to extend her 'experience' in an attempt to embrace the person's view of the care he receives and of his carer.

Four main relationships need to be examined. For reasons which are practical and logical we shall begin with the relationship which is furthest removed from the person in care. The nurse's relationship with her supervisor will be discussed first, since this is the primary relationship: the one which is happening in the 'here-and-now'. The nurse's relationship with the care plan will be considered next; followed by the nurse's relationship with herself, in terms of her 'use of self' in the caring process, and her personal reactions (reflections) on caring. The relationship with the person in care will be considered last since this was the starting point and is, therefore, furthest from the supervisory relationship currently operating.

## Nurse and Supervisor

Supervision which is not built upon an open, trusting, positive relationship will be virtually useless. Allocated supervisors should be aware of what, exactly, they are offering: is this an equal or a hierarchical relationship? The former will encourage exploration, discovery and growth; the latter will achieve more limited goals and may even foster dependency, or resentment. The supervisor–protégé relationship must begin with an examination of the underlying philosophy: 'Why are we meeting? What are our aims? What do we believe is important?' Once this is clarified, attention can turn to how the relationship might 'work'. If the nurse has not expressly selected her guide and mentor, then she needs to clarify what might be the limits of this supervisory relationship (or the limitations of her supervisor).

It has been noted earlier that the supervisor–protégé relationship reflects the clinical caring relationship. Both aim for growth and development, acceptance or adjustment. Practical details, such as how often sessions last, how often they take place, who defines the agenda and keeps the notes, etc., can be arranged with ease, possibly at the first meeting. Ritter (1989) provides detailed guidelines, comprising 23 'actions' with supporting rationales, which defines the practical process of supervision. Arranging means of communicating 'needs', expressing feelings, discussing 'taboo' topics, or simply exposing oneself to another may take much longer. Psychiatric problems are akin to icebergs. What do I do if I fear that the person I am working with at present is planning to kill himself. Do I tell my 'new' supervisor now, or do I simply review the 'tip' which is visible? The answer reveals the extent to which I trust my supervisor, if not also myself. The supervisor must not only demonstrate that she is trustworthy, but also that she can help the nurse trust herself.

How does such a relationship develop? This is a question similar to 'how long is a piece of string?'. My experience suggests that every supervisory relationship is different, since the pairings are different. What is common to them all is the need to maintain monitoring, a watching brief. Supervisor and protégé make a commitment when first they meet. This commits both parties to a policy of frankness, discipline and a mutual concern for the welfare of the person in care. Both parties need to review, at appropriate intervals, the development of their working relationship, checking on its healthiness and the general state of play. All relationships are characterized by three elements:

1. congruence, where both parties relate to one another on the basis of largely realistic pictures of themselves and each other;

2.  collusion, where both tacitly agree not to notice largely inaccurate self-conceptions in one or both of them; and
3.  contest, where one or both of them try to impose their definitions of themselves, or the other, on the other person.

Clearly, the hierarchical preceptor role described above reinforces contest, since the supervisor defines herself as the 'knowing' and the nurse as the 'ignorant'. Since this form of supervision is engineered, usually as part of an operational policy, there may also be a requirement for collusion. This is most likely where the 'learned' status of the supervisor is not readily apparent, but for organizational reasons must not be acknowledged.

Supervisors who are congruent will be the most successful and satisfying. Often this will involve them in losing themselves (i.e. temporarily turning away from their own values and personal concerns) by getting involved with the concerns of the protégé. Losing oneself in this manner projects an unconditional acceptance of the protégé (warts and all), and a willingness to share empathically her experience of care.

## Nurse and Care Plan

The supervisory process must include a critical appraisal of the care currently provided, with a view to amending or supplementing this, or changing direction completely. Although 'intellectual' in character, this examination involves the nurse's relationship with her work, which is an extension of herself. By its very nature this examination is potentially threatening and may raise issues and anxieties which will need to be addressed in the next part of the 'relationship'.

The supervisor encourages the nurse to assess the care plan at both a 'global' level, and in fine detail. In my view the critical features of all care plans are similar, irrespective of the setting in which care is conducted, or the population involved. The core features outlined in Table 5.1 can be used as the skeleton for this appraisal, examining the nurse's 'working relationship' with the person in care or significant others; her ability to organize the various stages of the care plan; her ability to identify and resolve problems met at any stage; and her use and understanding of the various technical aspects of care. Included here also are the nurse's description of the development and outcome of the care plan in whatever reporting format is considered appropriate.

The supervisor invites the nurse to describe the care plan to date, explaining what has been done and why. In addition to this 'subjective' evaluation by the nurse herself, the supervisor may also ask to see materials connected with the care plan, for example completed assessment charts, visual aids or record forms designed for use by staff or the

Table 5.1

| A. GENERAL | Rating | Comment |
|---|---|---|

1. Relationship with person
2. Relationship with significant others
3. Organization of care
4. Problem solving

| B. ASSESSMENT | | |
|---|---|---|

1. Selection
2. Handling
3. Guidelines
4. Rationale
5. Expectations/Orientation

| C. PLAN | | |
|---|---|---|

1. Identification of aims
2. Identification of sub-goals
3. Guidelines
4. Rationale
5. Selection of methods
6. Selection of monitoring method

| D. PROGRESS | | |
|---|---|---|

1. Structure and organization
2. Implementation
3. Evaluation
4. Adaptation and modification

| E. REPORTING | | |
|---|---|---|

1. Content
2. Style
3. Presentation

person himself, diaries, notes, graphs and other summary charts, as well as progress notes. The supervisor may consider it appropriate to sample the care process more directly by 'sitting in' on selected sessions, providing that this is agreeable to both the nurse and the person himself. Alternatively, the supervisor may ask the nurse to audio-tape sample interactions, with the same ethical proviso, to add a further dimension to the profile of the care process.

Some supervisors advocate making discrete judgements, in the form of ratings, of the various elements involved in the care plan (Barker, 1987). Ideally, both nurse and supervisor should judge the elements comprising Table 5.1, comparing their ratings and associated comments afterwards. Such a procedure encourages critical self-examination (from the nurse's perspective) whilst encouraging supervisors to be specific about perceived assets and deficits within the overall care plan. My experience suggests that emphasis upon the supervisor's 'objective' evaluation of the care plan can be transferred gradually to the nurse's subjective assessment of her own work. The supervisor's feedback helps the nurse reinforce her awareness of specific areas of competence or deficiency. The nurse is given an opportunity to look at her work initially through her supervisor's eyes, as a stepping stone towards a more objective self-examination (if that is not a contradiction in terms).

Although all aspects of the care plan are important, some elements might be seen as more vital than others. Supervisors may wish to focus more attention on areas such as confidentiality, ethical issues, the management of medication and other medical treatments, such as ECT, the person's role in the care plan (consent), and problems involving the safety of the person, other patients or the nurse's colleagues.

## Nurse and Self

The nurse's relationship with herself focuses mainly upon her expectations of what she should be doing, or her view of what she has already done. This appraisal considers what demands the care setting makes of the nurse. This can range from concerns about her work environment, workload, shift systems, noise, irregularities in circadian rhythms, demands on sleep–wakefulness, and so on, all of which can be stressful. The nurse needs an opportunity to review, comment, even simply to complain about coping with these pressures. In some cases the supervisor might consider it appropriate to encourage the nurse to suggest and experiment with possible 'solutions' using a negotiated timescale.

Consideration is also given to the demands she makes of herself. Some nurses find it difficult to cope with changes which they are required to make 'within themselves' in order to fulfil the person's needs. In others, the very nature of decision making and taking responsibility for specific individuals, acting as a primary nurse or keyworker, will bring their own pressures. Her 'failure' to respond to these demands may prove emotionally distressing. It is one of the supervisor's tasks to determine whether the source of any stress lies within the organization, or within the individual nurse (Hare, Pratt and Andrews, 1988). Unnecessary environmental stresses can be removed or reduced. Poor work rotas, inadequate equipment, lack of physical and moral support, all can be 'fixed', with a resultant reduction of stress. Where the stress lies in the nurse's 'use of self', the adjustment must be made on a personal level.

In psychiatric care much attention needs to be paid to the nurse's personal expectations. If she believes she should be able to help everyone towards successful rehabilitation or 'full growth', failure to achieve such lofty aims will be distressing. Where she is working with people who try to kill themselves, who reject her help, or who are dying or deteriorating from some physical cause (as with the confused elderly), her inability to help may generate strong feelings of guilt (Carder and Hall, 1981). Negative emotions which are experienced in such situations need to be acknowledged openly (Pryser, 1984). Although this appraisal ties in closely with the analysis of care goals and outcome mentioned above, specific attention needs to be paid here to the nurse's beliefs and feelings about 'cure' and 'rehabilitation'. What does she think is a 'good result'? The supervisor should be aware that 'psychic stress' is more likely where the person in care is regressed, aggressive, unmotivated, dependent, resistive or in some way 'incurable' (Vanderpool, 1984).

Care needs to be taken not to add to the nurse's difficulties by being too confrontational. The supervisor should be aware of the risk that the nurse might disguise or deny her fears and anxieties, or stifle feelings of frustration, interpreting these as signs of her own failure (Parkes, 1972). She may fear admitting such failings to her supervisor, especially if she appears to be a 'masterly' practitioner. The supervisor may need to model her own 'human frailty', by disclosing examples of her own fears, anxieties and frustrations, drawn from her own clinical experience. (From this perspective, supervision of one clinical nurse by another practitioner is almost essential.) The need to use disclosure, to facilitate sharing of common negative feelings, may be greatest in care of people with chronic mental disorder (Firth *et al.*, 1987; Jones *et al.*, 1987) or severe dementia (Athlin and Norberg, 1987). In either of these cases the nurse might feel that she should only experience positive feelings towards such 'unfortunates'. Her very real experiences of anger, frustration (or even fear and loathing of certain individuals) will generate extreme guilt. If properly accessed, clarified and discussed, the nurse may be able to accept such feelings as a natural part of the experience of caring.

## Nurse and Person in Care

The nurse's relationship with the person in care must emphasize 'personal' characteristics over 'clinical' considerations. If the nurse is inexperienced and apprehensive about the supervisory process, fairly focused questioning might enable her to begin framing a picture of what has happened so far in this relationship, as a basis for drawing upon her more subjective feelings: 'How often have you seen him?' 'Where do you meet?' 'For how long?' 'What have you discussed?' These pointed enquiries lead to more open-ended, general questions designed to allow the nurse more freedom to choose both the content focus and the emphasis she wishes to give. This 'wide-angle' focus is the starting point for the nurse with more experience of supervision. Typical opening questions might include:

'So how did you find Mr J . . .?' (inviting direct observation).
'How do you think your work with Mr J . . . is going?' (inviting intellectual reflection).
'How do you feel about this man?' (inviting emotional reflection).
'How do you think he feels about you, so far?' (inviting empathic statement).

This relationship underpins the three relationships already discussed. All of them are involved in a kind of dance. The nurse tries to identify the direction in which the person is moving; What needs is he pursuing? Where is he going? She tries to follow him, responding to things he says or does, sometimes in an attempt to be 'helpful', at others to 'help' him progress further in the required direction. Her actions will often prompt certain responses, encouraging him to do things, embrace certain ideas or even try to manipulate certain emotions. Supervision focuses upon what exactly is happening in this relationship. If, for example, the person describes himself as 'depressed' this description is not so much a statement of a natural emotion, as the application of a technical label, previously 'learned' by the person. The nurse needs to establish early on what this means. The person might then describe feelings of 'hopeless-ness', which in turn breed despair, lethargy and thoughts of suicide. The nurse's response to these sentiments has a major bearing on the developing relationship. Does she challenge this 'defeatist' talk, or does she encourage further exploration and reflection. The nurse who tries to draw the person 'back to reality' (as she understands it) too quickly, might simply advance the retreat being undertaken. Alternatively, the nurse who facilitates further discussion of these feelings, might serve as a prop, encouraging forward movement on the part of the person. The supervisor's role is to help the nurse to clarify how she sees the person, and to consider what he might see in her. At the same time consideration of the relationship triad, congruence, collusion and contest, might help her appreciate not only what is happening, but also what needs to be done.

**CONCLUSION**

Supervision is an emerging trend in nursing which will increase our chances of ensuring that 'quality' care is offered to everyone, and that as few nurses as possible suffer in the process. The contemporary view is that nursing needs to become more business-like. Those who manage services want to be able to measure the quality of care and want to know that financial cost is translated into effective care. This chapter has focused attention upon some nebulous issues which, I must confess, reflect my 20 years' experience of mental disorder and health. It is relatively easy to define and establish 'procedures', which are part and parcel of institutional life (see Ritter, 1989, for an excellent example). It is easy to operationalize the process for delivering anxiolytic medication. But what is the most 'effective' procedure for assessing whether this measure is necessary, how it will be received, and judging the alternatives? I am confident, also, in the belief that it is less easy to operationalize 'procedures' which might help people to feel valued, to confront their deeper anxieties, to live in the 'real world', or to share their lives with others. Organic nursing, like organic gardening, is a dirty business, and some people simply can't stand the smell.

This book is like hearing a welcome voice when lost in the dark. We are reassured, for the moment, but we know we can still become lost here, or somewhere else, again in the dark future. But still the reassurance is warmly accepted. Psychiatric nurses, at any stage of their professional development, are potentially vulnerable creatures. If they are to shed their professional uniformed cover, and 'get involved' with the people in their care at a human level, they risk exposing all their own human frailties and foibles. This may be too hot for some to handle. Ironically, many of the people who advocate the power of the 'interpersonal model' in nursing are no longer involved in relationships with 'patients'. I am thinking here especially of college-based tutors and nurse managers.

I want to see supervision on a grade scale within my own professional ranks. If we do not have it some people will 'burn out', and the rest will hide behind professional masks which people in care will, like Denton

Welch, find unpleasantly unhelpful. Supervision, providing that it is properly handled, might be the salvation of both the nurse and the person in care. The thread which I have tried to draw through this chapter represents a concern for welfare: the best interests of the person in care and of his carer. Hence my concern to protect people in care from nurses and nurses from themselves. Without supervision the 'quality nurse' will sacrifice herself for the best interests of her 'patient'; she will burn out. With supervision, we can have some guarantee of quality care without the risk of emotional life and limb.

I suspect that supervision will, for organizational reasons, become a prescribed commodity. This does not deflect me from my hoping that nurse and supervisor might share something akin to the close, mentoring relationship I have alluded to in this chapter. If they do not then psychiatric nurses may be able to learn a good many technical skills, but I fear that they will fail to grow any closer to the awareness of themselves and the nature of the calling of which they are a part. The activity of supervision in any area of nursing promises to reward the supervisor almost as much as it will the protégé. In psychiatric nursing, where the use and success of technical wizardry is less apparent, both mentor and protégé fall back on their intangible 'selves' for the content of both the caring and supervisory process. In psychiatric nursing, the use of self is the medium and the medium is the message.

## REFERENCES

Altschul, A. T. (1972) *Patient–nurse Interaction: A study of interactive patterns on acute psychiatric wards*, Churchill Livingstone, Edinburgh.
Athlin, E. and Norberg, A. (1987) Caregiver's attitudes to and interpretations of the behaviour of severely demented patients during feeding in a patient assignment care system. *International Journal of Nursing Studies*, **24**(2), 145–153.
Barker, P. (1987) Evaluation in nursing; The nurse as behaviour therapist, in *Evaluating Mental Health Practice: Methods and Applications* (Ed. D. Milne), Croom Helm, London.
Butterworth, C. A. (1987) Psychiatric nursing: Fumbling in a vacuum or grasping at opportunity. *Mental Health Nursing: The Journal of the Psychiatric Nurses Association*, October, 6.
Firth, H., McIntee, J., McKeown, P. and Britton, P. (1987) Professional depression, 'burnout' and personality in longstay nursing, *International Journal of Nursing Studies*, **24**(3), 227–237.
Carder, E. R. and Hall, C. V. (1981) The professional stress syndrome, *Psychosomatics*, **22**(8), 672.
Goffman, E. (1968) *Asylum: Essays on the social situation of mental patients and other inmates*, Penguin, Harmondsworth.

Hare, J., Pratt, C. C. and Andrew, D. (1988) Predictors of burnout in professional nurses working in hospitals and nursing homes, *International Journal of Nursing Studies*, **25**(2), 105–115.

Jones, G. J., Janman, K., Payne, R. L. and Rick, J. T. (1987) Some determinants of stress in psychiatric nursing, *International Journal of Nursing Studies*, **24**(2), 129–144.

Keith-Lucas, A. (1972) *Giving and Taking Help*, University of North Carolina Press, Chapel Hill.

Masson, J. (1989) *Against Therapy*, Collins, London.

Parkes, C. M. (1972) *Bereavement: studies of grief in adult life*, Penguin, Harmondsworth.

Peplau, H. (1986) Hildegard Peplau: Grande Dame of Psychiatric Nursing (interview), *Geriatric Nursing*, **7**(6), 328–330.

Pryser, P. (1984) Existential impact of professional exposure to life-threatening or terminal illness, *Bulletin of the Menninger Clinic*, **48**, 357–367.

Ritter, S. (1989) *Bethlem Royal and Maudsley Hospital Manual of Clinical Psychiatric Nursing Principles and Procedures*, Harper and Row, London.

Rowe, D. (1989) Foreword, *Against Therapy*, J. Masson, Collins, London.

Schwartz, M. S. and Shockley, E. L. (1956) *The Nurse and the Mental Patient: A study in interpersonal relations*, Russell Sage Foundation, New York.

Sullivan, H. S. (1947) *Conceptions of Modern Psychiatry*, William A. White, Psychiatric Foundation, Washington DC.

Travelbee, J. (1971) *Interpersonal Aspects of Nursing*, F. A. Davis, New York.

Vanderpool, J. P. (1984) Stressful patient relationships and the difficult patient, in *Rehabilitation Psychology* (Ed. P. N. Krueger), Aspen, Rockville, Md.

Welch, D. (1983) *A Voice Through a Cloud*, King Penguin, Harmondsworth.

# CHAPTER SIX

# Clinical supervision in sick children's nursing

*Barbara Elliott*

## INTRODUCTION

The nursing of sick children has been considered as separate and different from nursing adults throughout the profession's history. The Nurses Registration Act (1919) set up five separate parts to the Register of Nurses, one of these parts being that containing the names of nurses trained in the nursing of sick children (Ministry of Health, 1919). The care of sick children will continue to require separate educational preparation in the future as recognized by the establishment of children's nursing as one of the four specialist branches in Project 2000.

It is reasonable, therefore, that supervision of sick children's nurses be considered as being distinct from supervision of nurses in other specialties. This chapter will firstly consider supervision applied to the paediatric setting and then examine two of the major components which make sick children's nursing unique: play and the involvement of non-professionals (mainly parents) in care.

The chapter discusses supervision in sick children's nursing and therefore focuses on children nursed in paediatric wards and units, be they in a general hospital or paediatric hospital. It is realized that this is not always the case, with 25% of child in-patients being nursed on adult or mixed wards (Caring for Children in the Health Services, 1987).

## CLINICAL SUPERVISION

Pettes (1967) describes supervision as 'a process by which one practitioner is accountable to another practitioner to help him practise to the best of his ability'. This broad definition is desirable so as to encompass the many and varied forms of supervision in the clinical setting.

Supervision is most readily thought of in terms of education where 'the role of the supervisor is to respond to the perceived needs of the student or new recruit and to provide learning opportunities appropriate to those needs' (Jarvis, 1984, p. 126). The best person to fulfil the role of supervisor in this context has long been debated and many would agree with Kenworthy and Nicklin (1989) that the only credible and professionally acceptable person to function in this capacity is the practising nurse. This may be doing a great disservice to many experienced nurse tutors and clinical teachers who see their role in the supervision of students being eroded. However, practical limitations of time frequently necessitate nurse teachers passing on at least some of their supervisory role to ward staff.

Student nurses do not have a monopoly on the need for supervision. Any practitioner involved in a therapeutic relationship with a patient or client may find it difficult to step back and evaluate the effectiveness of that relationship. Supervision may provide the objective validation of the helping relationship and is of great importance to experienced practitioners as well as novices (Sundeen *et al.*, 1985). All nurses, including sick children's nurses, need a means of ensuring that they are supervised throughout their professional lives. Sick children's nurses, however, like other hospital-based nurses, have been slow to formalize the supervisory relationship for practitioners other than students. Supervision does exist within the paediatric setting, indeed it is essential for the maintenance and delivery of high standards of care. However, it has many forms and at times may be so subtle as to be almost undetectable.

Barber (1987) describes formal and informal supervision. The primary task of formal supervision is the supervision itself, but in informal supervision the primary task is the delivery of care. Informal supervision enables assessment of a nurse's capabilities in a less threatening manner than formal supervision. Nurses in charge of wards are responsible for allocating patient care to appropriate staff. It is therefore essential that they are aware of each staff member's level of ability and competence. This is usually discovered through a means of informal supervision. In sick children's nursing this informal supervision is more difficult to achieve because of the nature of care required. Nursing care of adult patients frequently requires two nurses: to bed bath, turn or lift a patient, for example. This gives the supervisor, be she ward sister, staff nurse or clinical teacher, an ideal opportunity to work with the supervisee in a non-threatening way. By assisting the supervisee the supervisor can assess her practical and interpersonal skills on which she can base future decisions about the types of patients she is best able to care for. The supervisor may later give the supervisee feedback on her performance and together they can identify areas to be developed.

Care of children, however, frequently requires only one nurse and the supervisor may feel awkward, having no other reason for being present than that she wishes to observe the nurse at work. With experience the supervisor may be able to ensure that her presence is not intrusive, but like the non-participant observer in research her very presence may make the situation unnatural and make the supervisee and patient feel ill at ease. There is a risk also that, in order to cope with her own feelings, the supervisor may take over completely. The junior student may welcome the opportunity to observe a competent role model, but the more experienced student or sick children's nurse may resent the inferred criticism of her ability and interference with her nursing care. An alternative to this one-to-one supervision is group supervision or peer review. This may take place at handover reports, ward meetings, group counselling sessions or multidisciplinary case conferences.

Ward meetings provide an excellent opportunity for general policies and standards to be discussed and staff may divulge individual problems. There is little evidence as yet however that such meetings formalize peer review or supervision.

Clinical case presentation as practised in community psychiatric nursing (Butterworth, 1988) has not been documented in sick children's nursing, but multidisciplinary meetings, where the care of individual or groups of patients is discussed, can be seen to have certain common characteristics. Such meetings are usually held to discuss children with the same or similar diseases and are aimed at combining information from different sources and encouraging a united approach to care. Treatment and progress is evaluated and each member of the health care team has an opportunity to discuss their individual contribution to care. This form of multidisciplinary supervision is very valuable and provides a means of objective evaluation for all levels of staff.

## SUPERVISION OF PLAY

One of the major differences between a children's and an adult ward is the noise and level of activity. Indeed the uninitiated are often amazed at the apparent chaos and commotion of a children's ward. This state of affairs is usually the result of play in its many forms.

Psychologists have examined the functions of play in childhood and each has her/his own perspective on its importance. For example Erickson (1940) considered play as one of the major ego functions and the means by which the child endeavours to organize his inner world in relation to his outer. Children learn to 'play out' their emotions, frustrations and sufferings and thus make sense of them. Piaget (1962) considered that the development of play was closely linked with the development of intelligence and described play as the medium of learning. Whatever the functions of play there is an agreement that, as well as being pleasurable and intensely absorbing, play is essential for the development of the child's physical, psychological and social functioning and well-being.

Children in hospital therefore must be encouraged to play in order to continue their normal development for as Wall states in Weller (1980), 'The child who cannot play is as severely threatened as the child who is deprived of nourishment'. For the child in hospital play may be the one normal element left in his world, which has otherwise been turned upside down.

> Like a stranger in a foreign country who suddenly hears his own language, the child reaches out to play in anticipation of friendship in a bewildering and frightening situation. Hott (1970, p. 307)

Play is also essential for the hospitalized child as a means of expressing his emotions and enabling him to make sense of what is happening to him. The effect of play on the psychological well-being of young children in hospital was studied by Noble (1967). She found that in wards where there was no special provision for play the children demonstrated most signs of disturbance. Petrillo and Sanger (1981) claim that play is one of the most powerful and effective means of stress reduction for children and emphasize its importance in hospitalization. This reduction in stress and anxiety through play has been associated with an increase in rate of recovery (Garot, 1986).

For children's nurses play is the means by which they can communicate with their young patients, gain their trust and encourage their cooperation (Weller, 1980; D'Antonio, 1984). Communication with sick children is essential in order to explain what is happening to them and what will happen in the future, in order to reduce their anxiety. Klinzing and Klinzing (1977) state that the primary reason for fear amongst hospitalized children is lack of understanding, but they warn that any means of providing information must take account of the child's intellectual ability.

The use of play in providing children with information about their hospital stay, medical and surgical procedures and helping them deal with their emotions has been frequently documented (Knudsen, 1975; Azarnoff and Flegal, 1975; Rodin, 1983; D'Antonio, 1984) and the benefits of play as a means of preparation are not disputed.

The ability to facilitate play and use it as a means of building a therapeutic relationship with her patient is a recognized skill of the sick children's nurse. Emphasis is placed on the importance of play during training for registration as a sick children's nurse (English National Board, 1982). However, like talking to adult patients, play is often given low priority and is only to be indulged in after the 'work' is completed. Nurses may be frequently called away from playing in order to carry out clinical duties and it is now recognized that the

> special functions of play in the life of the child in hospital cannot be achieved unless an appropriately trained play specialist is present and unless the play specialist is working as an integral member of the paediatric team. (Save the Children, 1989, p. 30)

This statement follows many years of striving to give play the status it deserves. The first official recognition of the need for play for children in hospital was made as part of the Platt Report (Ministry of Health, 1959). The recommendations of this report regarding play were not generally implemented by hospitals and the setting up of play schemes was mainly left to voluntary organizations such as Save the Children Fund, the National Association for the Welfare of Children in Hospital (NAWCH) and the Preschool Playgroups Association (PPA). Some health authorities did set up their own play schemes and others took over the running of the schemes once the voluntary agencies had set them up.

Recognizing the importance of play for children in hospital and the need for more hospital play schemes the DHSS Expert Group on Play for Children in Hospital (1976) considered it unrealistic to expect nurses to take on total responsibility for play and recommended that play workers be appointed in all children's wards. The DHSS while accepting the therapeutic advantage of encouraging play among children in hospital, rejected the advice of their Expert Group on Play and suggested instead that play should become part of nurses' work with children and that nurses should be given special training to this end.

Until this time the clinical model had dominated nurse training and the emphasis of nursing care was very much on the physical care of child patients, keeping the wards neat and tidy and minimizing noise (Hawthorn, 1974).

Studies of children's nursing in the 1960s and 1970s repeatedly showed that nurses spent a very small amount of their time playing with their young patients (Pill, 1970; Hawthorn, 1974). Pill (1970) found that the nurses in her study did not perceive their role as including playing with or talking to the children on their ward. The time that an individual child spent interacting with the nurses was on average half an hour, the majority of interactions being when the nurse was engaged in basic nursing care.

Hawthorn (1974) found that the hospitalized children in her study were alone and awake for a large amount of time and that there was a fundamental lack of knowledge among nursing staff of the emotional needs of the children. She recommended that there was an urgent need for senior nursing staff in paediatric wards to be given the opportunity to learn about current child care theories.

The lack of involvement of nurses in play was reflected as late as 1983 in Rodin's valuable work, which examined the benefits of preparing children for having blood taken by venepuncture. She sought to find a method of play preparation which could be used by parents and children unaided. Her review of the literature had revealed that previous preparation schemes were limited because they demanded too much time from busy hospital personnel and that parents were often the best people to prepare their children. Whilst not disputing the last fact it is a sad reflection of the low priority given to play by nurses that they did not value their own involvement in play schemes.

The introduction of play workers to children's wards has improved the opportunities for sick children to play, however their acceptance by nursing colleagues and the utilization of their special skills and knowledge has not been an automatic result. Hall (1977) studied the effects of the introduction of a play leader to two general acute hospitals in Great Britain. He found that they enabled the children to have greater freedom of movement and activity in the wards. However the nursing staff were reluctant to give the play leaders much medical information and thus maintained a distinction between the care of sick children in the ward and the occupation of less ill children in the play room. The nurses therefore failed to fully utilize the play leaders' skills. They unanimously agreed that play was a part of their, the nurses, duties, but observation suggested that when they were busy it was one of their lowest priorities and when they were less busy they did not possess the knowledge or experience to be able to perform the role.

The situation today is much improved. The focus of play workers has changed from mother substitute to play therapist and it is recommended that Health Authorities employ staff with the national qualification offered by the Hospital Play Staff Examination Board (Save the Children, 1989). However the career structure of play workers remains limited with no standardized structure for pay and conditions and no universally accepted title.

This background to the employment and status of play and play workers in paediatric wards has implications for the clinical supervision of sick children's nurses. Today many paediatric wards employ a play worker, although the last survey of play in hospital carried out by the Play in Hospital Liaison Committee and Save the Children Fund in 1985 revealed that the number was nowhere near that recommended with only 37.02% of wards admitting more than 50 children per annum having a salaried play worker. It is even more essential therefore that where they do exist the experience and knowledge of the play workers is fully utilized.

It has recently been recommended that play specialists should be involved in the training of hospital staff about the needs of children and adolescents (Hogg, 1990). This may be seen as the first step towards official recognition of the teaching potential of play workers. Their potential for supervision is also just being realized and it is to be hoped that professional jealousies and an adherence to the strict hierarchy of supervision will not prevent sick children's nurses from taking full advantage of the play leaders' expertise.

Hall (1977) found that there was no evidence that nurses could learn from the play workers' example without instructions or encouragement from supervisors. Thus it would seem that the play leaders' authority needs official recognition from senior nurses and managers before less experienced nurses can learn from them. More recent publications (Save the Children, 1989; Hogg, 1990) stress the need for the role of the play specialist to be seen as a professional one, independent of, but complementary to, other members of the health care team. Such a change in status may assist play specialists to take on a supervisory role for junior or inexperienced nursing staff.

If we are to accept that the most credible and professionally acceptable person to teach is the person directly involved in care (Kenworthy and Nicklin, 1989) then perhaps it is time that play workers be recognized as the best people to teach and supervise play. Nurses are developing their teaching and assessing skills to meet the needs of their students (notably the development of the ENB course 998, Teaching and Assessing in Clinical Practice) and perhaps similar opportunities should be extended to play staff.

Recognizing the two-way relationship of supervision, play workers also need someone who can objectively assess their effectiveness with a patient. Play therapy is increasingly being used with children who have behavioural or emotional problems and this can involve the play worker in a very intense relationship with the child. Although such play staff will have received special training for this job, they nevertheless need supervision to evaluate their relationship and discuss possible initiatives and progress. It is recommended that hospitals employ a senior play specialist to coordinate play staff (Hogg, 1990) and they could take on some of this supervisory role. However it is unlikely that, if employed at all, such a person would be able to provide regular supervision for all play staff. In practice the relative isolation and lack of career structure within their own profession means that play workers frequently rely on sick children's nurses to fulfil this role.

The role of supervision in play is as yet undeveloped. If it is accepted that play is an important part of the sick children's nurses role then responsibility must be taken for supervising nurses in this capacity. In many respects there has been little progress since Hall's observations (1977) in that frequently play is viewed as a job for junior or untrained nurses, and is seen as a means of entertaining the children and preventing boredom. The old expression 'he is only playing' as applied to children may well be applied to the attitude often expressed toward nurses involved in play. The implication that play is indulged in by those with nothing better to do is unforgivable. The vital role that play has in the care and treatment of sick children must be recognized. Supervision of play may then be given the priority it deserves.

## PARENTAL PARTICIPATION IN CARE

In few areas of nursing are non-professionals so closely involved in care as in paediatrics. As long ago as 1927 Spence was admitting mothers with their sick babies to hospital in Newcastle, but it was not until the 1950s that the possible harmful effects of separation of children from their parents first began to be highlighted. Bowlby's (1951) work on maternal deprivation was supported by that of James Robertson, who in 1953 produced the evocative film 'A Two Year Old goes into Hospital' which brought realization to the general public that 'the greatest single cause of distress to young children in hospital is not pain or illness, but separation from mother' (Robertson, 1953).

The evidence of Robertson (1958) to the Platt Committee, established by the Ministry of Health to look at the welfare of children in hospital, was very influential in establishing the recommendations of the Committee. The Platt Report (Ministry of Health, 1959) recommended amongst other things unrestricted parental visiting and the provision of accommodation for mothers of sick children, especially those under five years. The hospitals were slow to implement government recommendations and the National Association for the Welfare of Children in Hospital (NAWCH) was set up in 1961 to promote their implementation.

Those hospitals that did allow parents free access to their sick children did not encourage them to be involved in care. This caused mothers to feel frustrated, bored and unsure of how much they were allowed to do for their child (Meadow, 1969; Webb, 1977). The nurses did not feel helped by the mother's presence, as was presumed by the Platt Committee, but indeed they felt hindered in their work.

Whilst taking account of the psychological evidence the Platt

Committee had not received or considered sociological evidence. The implications of their recommendations on the social situations of the hospital, the roles of the nursing and medical staff and their relationships with parents had been insufficiently recognized (Hall, 1978).

Initially nurses continued to care for children as if the mothers were not there, often refusing or ignoring their offers of help (Stacey *et al.*, 1970). Gradually the situation has changed, although there is still no general consensus amongst children's nurses about the extent or form of parental participation. Parents are increasingly encouraged on most wards to continue the normal care that they would give to their child at home during a hospital admission. This includes care given to meet the everyday needs of the child, such as bathing, dressing and feeding. Such care would obviously be given by a nurse if the child's parents were absent or unable to continue their normal child care.

This care, often termed 'family care', may be all the parents are willing or able to do and no pressure should be put upon them to do more. However, parents are increasingly learning to give nursing care, that is care relating to the health needs of the child, such as giving nasogastric feeds, tracheostomy care and changing dressings. Involvement of parents in nursing care is seen as a natural progression and of benefit to children, parents, medical and nursing staff (Webb, Hull and Madeley, 1985; Sainsbury *et al.*, 1986; Bishop, 1988; Goodwin, 1988; Taylor and O'Connor, 1989). This assumption that parental participation in care is desirable reflects the changing expectations and attitudes amongst health care professionals towards the role of the parent in the care of the sick child.

The relationship between that care which is given by the sick children's nurse and that which is given by the parents is often in a delicate balance. The nurse must carefully negotiate with parents the care that they wish to give and feel confident giving, that care which they require help with, the nursing care which they would like to learn to give and the care which they would never be happy giving under any circumstances. The nurse must be wary of leaving the parent to give 'family care' unsupervised when the child's condition means that their normal competence and confidence is impaired. Such a situation might be leaving the parent to dress a child who has an intravenous infusion. Similarly the nurse must be wary of coercing parents into learning to give nursing care when they already feel frightened and unsure about giving their usual family care.

Attempts are being made to formalize this relationship in terms of developing a model of nursing which incorporates parental and nursing interventions (Casey, 1988). The essential ingredients of this relationship must be communication and partnership. Knafl and Dixon (1984), following their analysis of fathers' participation in their children's hospitalization, concluded that it was essential that nurses openly discussed with parents their respective roles and the degree of parental participation desired.

This situation of non-professionals delivering care to the sick child, be it family or nursing care, has implications for clinical supervision in sick children's nursing. These implications will be considered in two sections: parents as supervisors and supervising parents.

## PARENTS AS SUPERVISORS

In most situations the sick child's parents may be regarded as the experts in family care. They know their child better than anyone else, they know his likes and dislikes, his normal routines and favourite games. A junior nurse may feel threatened by an experienced, confident mother, but who better to supervise her in learning new skills of family care than that expert mother? Junior nurses should be encouraged to work as partners with parents, to learn from them and accept their unique knowledge of their child. Parents can usually see through a nurse's pretence at being experienced in child care when she is not, and would feel much more confident in entrusting their child's care to a nurse whom they have already supervised giving that care. Even the experienced nurse will benefit from working with the child's parents so that she can continue to do things 'just like mummy does them', should the parents have to leave. It is unrealistic to expect parents to keep a constant vigil by their child's bedside, but occasionally parents dare not leave, even for a cup of coffee, because they fear that no-one will know what to do if their child cries.

The situation is often more apparent with children with physical and/or mental disabilities. The parents of these children are often already experts in aspects of nursing care and cope by having regular routines for such problems as elimination. Their child may have difficulties in communicating his needs and the parents have to become experts in interpreting facial expressions, movements or sounds. When such children are admitted to hospital, particularly if it is an unfamiliar ward, there may be role conflicts between their families and nurses. Ferraro and Longo (1985) suggest that these role conflicts are caused by the competency and confidence which families have developed through caring for their sick child and the usual model of care for acutely ill children encountered on the ward. It may be asserted that these very competent mothers prefer to continue giving all of their child's care and the nurse may take on a passive role. This may well be so, but it may also be that the parents do not trust the nurses to deliver care of an equal standard in their absence. If these parents were encouraged to spend a few hours supervising a sick children's nurse caring for their child they might then

feel confident enough to take a much needed break whilst their child is in
hospital.

Parents who are taught to give technical nursing or medical care, such
as intravenous drug administration, are taught the very high standards
demanded by hospital protocols. They become technical experts, their
technique having to be so continually perfect as to ensure that, on
discharge, standards are not lowered. On subsequent hospital admissions
the care may be taken over for a short period by medical or nursing staff,
which may lead to problems. Doctors in particular may be unaware of the
parents' knowledge and skills and may become indignant if their
technique is criticized by the parents. Parents supervising care in this
manner may be seen as threatening by staff, but in fact it can ensure
scrupulous adherence to correct procedure and policy.

It is noteworthy that children receiving long-term treatment also
become experts in their own care. They may not be able to undertake the
care themselves, but quietly supervise the hospital staff. The hesitant,
unconfident or inexperienced practitioner is soon exposed by children
who are not reticent in telling a doctor or nurse when they are not
performing skills to the required standard!

## SUPERVISING PARENTS

Many children are admitted to hospital because the family care given by
parents is not of a sufficiently high standard to prevent ill health or they
require nursing or medical care to meet their health needs. Parents will
then need careful assessment of their capabilities and learning needs. If
parents are to contribute to the care of their sick child, the level of their
contribution must be decided as described earlier and a programme of
education and supervision devised. This may involve supervising family
care, such as the sterilization of feeding equipment for a young baby, or
nursing care, such as the management of a raised temperature. Sick
children's nurses need to use all their counselling and supervisory skills to
enable parents to develop their full potential.

In some 'care by parents' schemes, such as that described by Cleary *et
al.* (1986), the nurse's main function is to teach, support and counsel
parents who deliver and record all their child's care. Such schemes have
been very successful in terms of reducing the time the children are alone
and awake or crying and ensuring that the majority of their contacts are
with a family member, usually their mother (Cleary *et al.*, 1986). Medical
and nursing staff have also found such schemes satisfactory, but to date
they have been slow to develop in this country.

The role of parents in the care of sick children will continue to
develop. Sick children's nurses must therefore continue to reassess their

role with parents and be prepared to accept supervision from parents and in return give such supervision to them as the changing situation demands.

## CONCLUSION

Sick children are not miniature sick adults: they have their own unique problems and needs and their nursing care requires skills quite different from those required for nursing adults. In this chapter, two areas in sick children's nursing have been discussed which require specialist skills and education for practising nurses and raise issues regarding clinical supervision for those nurses. An attempt has been made to address some of those issues and suggestions made for the future of clinical supervision in sick children's nursing. There are of course many other aspects to this specialist area of nursing and the implementation of Project 2000 and the future development of primary nursing and sick children's community nursing services will provide further areas for consideration.

Sick children's nursing is at an exciting point in its development. Whatever the future holds, children will continue to have special needs, and supervision of their nursing care will play a major role in ensuring that those needs are met.

## REFERENCES

Azarnoff, P. and Flegal, S. (1975) *A Paediatric Play Programme*, Charles C. Thomas, Illinois.
Barber, P. (1987) Skills in supervision, *Nursing Times*, 14 Jan., 56–57.
Bishop, J. (1988) Sharing the caring, *Nursing Times*, **84**(30), 60–61.
Bowlby, J. (1951) *Maternal Care and Mental Health*, Geneva, World Health Organisation.
Butterworth, C. (1988) Breaking the boundaries, *Nursing Times and Nursing Mirror*, **84**, 23 Nov., 36–39.
Caring for Children in the Health Services (1987) *Where are the Children?*, NAWCH, London.
Casey, A. (1988) A partnership with child and family, *Senior Nurse*, **8**(4), 8–9.
Cleary, J., Gray, O. P., Hall, D. J. *et al.* (1986) Parental involvement in the lives of children in hospital, *Archives of Disease in Childhood*, **61**, 770–787.
D'Antonio, I. J. (1984) Therapeutic use of play in hospitals, *Nursing Clinics of North America*, **19**(2), 351–359.
DHSS (1976) *The Report of the Expert Group on Play in Hospital*, HMSO, London.
English National Board (1982) *Aspects of Sick Children's Nursing – A Learning Package*, London.

Erickson, E. H. (1940) Studies in the interpretation of play, *Genet. Psychol. Monograph*, **22**, 561.

Ferraro, A. R. and Longo, D. C. (1985) Nursing care of the family with a chronically ill, hospitalised child. An alternative approach, *Image*, **17**(2), 77–81.

Goodwin, P. (1988) 'I know you're busy but . . .', *Nursing Times*, **84**(30), 62.

Hall, D. J. (1977) *Social Relations and Innovation Changing the State of Play in Hospitals*, Routledge and Kegan Paul, London.

Hall, D. J. (1978) Bedside blues: The impact of social research on the hospital treatment of sick children, *Journal of Advanced Nursing*, **3**(1), 25–37.

Hawthorn, P. (1974) *Nurse – I Want My Mummy*, Royal College of Nursing, London.

Hott, J. (1970) Play P.R.N. in paediatric nursing, *Nursing Forum*, **IX**(3), 288–309.

Jarvis, P. (1984) The educational role of the supervisor in the tutorial relationship, *Nurse Education Today*, **3**(6), 126–129.

Kenworthy, N. and Nicklin, P. (1989) *Teaching and Assessing in Nursing Practice, An Experiential Approach*, Scutari Press, London.

Klinzing, D. R. and Klinzing, R. G. (1977) *The Hospitalised Child Communication Techniques for Health Personnel*, Prentice-Hall, New Jersey.

Knafl, K. A. and Dixon, D. (1984) The participation of fathers in their children's hospitalisation, *Issues in Comprehensive Paediatric Nursing*, **7**, 269–281.

Knudsen, K. (1975) Play therapy, preparing the young child for surgery, *Nursing Clinics of North America*, **10**(1), 679–686.

Meadow, S. R. (1969) The captive mother, *Archives of Disease in Childhood*, **44**, 363–367.

Ministry of Health for England and Wales (1919) *Nurses Registration Act*, HMSO, London.

Ministry of Health (1959) *The Welfare of Children in Hospital (the Platt Report)*, HMSO, London.

National Association for the Welfare of Children in Hospital (1984) *NAWCH Charter for Children in Hospital*, NAWCH, London.

Noble, E. (1967) *Play and the Sick Child*, Faber, London.

Pettes, D. E. (1967) *Supervision in Social Work: A Method of Student Training and Staff Development*, National Institute for Social Work Training, Series Number 10, Allen and Unwin, London.

Petrillo, M. and Sanger, S. (1972) *Emotional Care of Hospitalised Children*, Lippincott, Philadelphia.

Piaget, J. (1962) *Play, Dreams and Limitation in Childhood*, W. W. Norton and Co., New York.

Pill, R. (1970) The sociological aspects of the case study sample, in *Hospitals, Children and Their Families* (Ed. M. Stacey), Routledge and Kegan Paul, London.

Robertson, J. (1953) *A Two Year Old Goes To Hospital* (A Scientific Film Record), Tavistock Clinic for Human Relations, London.

Robertson, J. (1958) *Young Children in Hospital*, Tavistock Publications Ltd., London.

Rodin, J. (1983) *Will This Hurt? Preparing Children for Hospital and Medical Procedures*, Royal College of Nursing, London.

Sainsbury, C. P. Q., Gray, O. P., Cleary, J. *et al.* (1986) Care by parents of their children in hospital, *Archives of Disease in Childhood*, **61**, 612–615.

Stacey, M., Dearden, R., Pill, R. and Robinson, D. (1970) *Hospitals, Children and their Families*, Routledge and Kegan Paul, London.

Sundeen, S. J., Stuart, G. W., Rankin, E. and Cohen, S. (1985) *Nurse Client Interaction*, Mosby, St Louis.

Taylor, M. R. H. and O'Connor, P. (1989) Resident parents and shorter hospital stay, *Archives of Disease in Childhood*, **64**(2), 274–276.

Webb, B. (1977) Trauma and tedium: An account of living in on a children's ward, in *Medical Encounters* (Ed. A. Davies and G. Horobin), Croom Helm, London.

Webb, N., Hull, D. and Madeley, R. (1985) Care by parents in hospital, *British Medical Journal*, **291**, 176–177.

Weller, B. F. (1980) *Helping Sick Children Play*, Baillière Tindall, London.

# CHAPTER SEVEN

# Supervision in clinical midwifery practice

*Penny Curtis*

> This was not just Mary Cronk being told to give syntometrine in the Isle of Wight: it was something that was absolutely basic to a midwife's right to practise.
>
> This hospital policy is binding on all midwives once they cross the threshold of a hospital. If we are employed in the hospital to practise according to hospital policy we are no longer midwives. We are no longer practitioners. (MIDIRS, 1987)

In 1987, a community midwife practising in the Isle of Wight aroused considerable interest in the professional press (Flint, 1987; Hughes and Parker, 1987; *Nursing Times*, 1987), when she contested the right of her midwifery manager and supervisor of midwives to direct her clinical practice. Her supervisor of midwives had issued a memorandum directing all midwives who conducted hospital deliveries to administer syntometrine for the third stage of labour (unless the mother gave specific instructions to the contrary). The directive had been originated by a consultant obstetrician.

Many midwives will be familiar with the situation that Mary Cronk describes.

> I encountered this in the field of episiotomies: *all* women will have episiotomies, I have recently encountered it in the last few years: all women will have their membranes ruptured. I said on both these occasions if in my clinical judgement it is necessary, yes I will make an episiotomy and if in my clinical judgement it is not necessary I will not make an episiotomy. If I think an amniotomy is indicated I will make an amniotomy; if I don't think an amniotomy is necessary I won't make an amniotomy. I think the same thing pertains to the

management of the first stage of labour or any other management of a parturient woman and her baby. (MIDIRS, 1987)

The Isle of Wight midwives' affair illustrates very concisely the conflicts that midwives experience at work. Mary Cronk made a stand in support of a fundamental right, the right to control her own work. If we hope to analyse midwives' experience of midwifery with any degree of sensitivity, we must recognize at the outset that the statutory supervision of midwifery as it is embodied in the rules and regulations, and the code of professional conduct, cannot on its own offer a comprehensive insight into their work. Formal professional control delineates midwifery *vis à vis* other occupations. To those outside (as well as inside) the profession, it defines who can justly call herself (1) a midwife and the boundaries within which she can work. The statutory structure functions both to protect the public from incompetent or negligent practitioners, and to protect the practitioner from the public. However, because midwifery has a statutory system of supervision it is easy to be swayed by the conspicuousness of the formal structures and to fail to recognize the importance of informal supervision.

In this chapter I will focus for the most part upon the complex web of informal social relationships which, although largely unseen by persons outside of the immediate work setting, has a very real influence upon clinical practice, and upon the midwife's daily experience of work. However, a brief consideration of the formal supervisory structure is a necessary prerequisite in order to develop a feel for the way in which formal supervision impinges upon the midwife's working day.

The definition of a midwife adopted by the International Confederation of Midwives and the International Federation of Gynaecologists and Obstetricians reads as follows:

A midwife is a person who, having been regularly admitted to a midwifery educational programme, duly recognised in the country in which it is located, has successfully completed the prescribed course of studies in midwifery and has acquired the requisite qualifications to be registered and/or legally licensed to practise midwifery.

She must be able to give the necessary supervision, care and advice to women during pregnancy, labour and the postpartum period, to conduct deliveries on her own responsibility and to care for the newborn and the infant. This care includes preventative measures, the detection of abnormal conditions in mother and child, the procurement of medical assistance and the execution of emergency measures in the absence of medical help. She has an important task in health counselling and education, not only for the patients, but also within the family and the community. The work should involve antenatal education and preparation for parenthood and extends to certain areas of gynaecology, family planning and child care. She may practise in hospitals, clinics, health units, domiciliary conditions or in any other service (UKCC, 1986a).

The profession's governing body is the United Kingdom Central Council for Nursing, Midwifery and Health Visiting. However, while the statutory rules for the regulation of midwives and midwifery practice are framed by the UKCC (functioning in accordance with the recommendations of its midwifery committee) these rules and regulations, and the code of professional conduct have not, of course, developed in a vacuum but have arisen out of a set of social relations. As such, they reflect the conflicts and compromises worked out between powerful interest groups. In particular, the authority of the higher status medical profession has been formalized and built into the profession's rules and regulations. Contemporary midwifery knowledge and authority is qualified. The midwife is the expert in 'normal' midwifery who, at the same time, is bound 'to carry out the treatment prescribed by a doctor' (Article 4:10 of the European Community Midwives' Directive 80/155/EEC, which defines the activities that midwives are entitled to take up and pursue). The UKCC also draws up rules concerning the training of midwives and maintains the professional register, as indeed it does for all areas of nursing and health visiting. The Board is the pinnacle, the distant head of the hierarchical structure of statutory supervision as it affects the practising midwife.

On the next layer, each of the four National Boards collects notices of intention to practise from each local supervising authority, approves training institutions and is responsible for the investigation of cases of alleged misconduct or ill health. General responsibility for the supervision of all midwives practising in their area is delegated to LSA's (local supervising authorities), regional health authorities in England, district health authorities in Wales, health boards in Scotland and health and social services boards in Northern Ireland. The LSAs are guided by their respective National Boards. The LSAs are responsible for reporting cases of professional misconduct to the National Boards, and have the power to suspend midwives from practice.

At the base of this hierarchical structure is situated the supervisor of midwives. She is appointed by the local supervising authority to provide supervision of midwifery practice in each health authority, unit or sub-unit. The supervisor of midwives personifies the formal supervisory structure. She is required to bring the distant professional hierarchy to bear upon the daily practice of clinical midwifery. However, since its inception, supervision has been tied into and compromised by the administrative structure. Today, the midwives' supervisory machinery operates through the bureaucratic structures of the National Health Service in which the majority of midwives are employed. In addition, although supervisors of midwives must be registered midwives with clinical midwifery experience, appointees are 'normally the senior midwifery managers within health authorities' (UKCC, 1986a), midwives who have moved away from a clinical role.

Individual post holders face contradictory expectations as agents of management who are simultaneously expected to be a source of professional support and guidance to whom the practitioner is advised to turn 'on all matters as required by the Midwife's Practice Rules and [the] Code of Practice and on any other matter on which she may need help or advice' (UKCC, 1986b). The contradictions imbued in the supervisor of midwives' role have recently aroused comment in the midwifery press, and have led some midwives to suggest that clinical supervision should be divorced from managerial control (Isherwood, 1988). Walker illustrates this sentiment:

In particular, I feel supervisors of midwives should be practising, experienced midwives who are respected by their peers and should *not* be managers. There are always great difficulties when a supervisor is a manager who is continually being harassed by general managers to cope under the pressures of this present difficult time and many cannot divide the two roles.

I want my supervisor of midwives to be my guide, counsellor and friend. A practising midwife I respect. (Walker, 1988)

The embodiment of statutory supervisory responsibility in individuals employed as agents of management confuses bureaucratic and professional control and influences the way in which midwives perceive formal supervision. The statutory structure appears remote to the midwife on the ground. Formal supervision is conceived of in terms of large, extrinsic issues which have a limited bearing upon the interpersonal relations that are part and parcel of daily work. Warren (1988) suggests that

I know of many midwives who are more scared of their local managers or Supervisors of Midwifery than the possible consequences of ignoring the Midwives Rules or the Code of Professional Conduct.

The rules and regulations of the statutory supervisory structure enable us to envisage the parameters within which midwives work, but the hard and fast image that they portray is misleading. To look inside these parameters, to understand the midwife's occupational room to manoeuvre, we also need to consider the informal processes of clinical supervision that develop as a response to the constraints that midwives experience in their daily practice. At this point it is worthwhile setting down an essential truism: midwifery, like any other form of work, is more than the performance of physical tasks. Midwives also experience and reproduce social relations as part of their daily work. Through ongoing processes of interaction a fluid plexus of informal relationships is built up as part of a dynamic workplace culture. Supervisory relationships are integral elements of the cultural milieu that evolves in each clinical setting. Informal or invisible processes confound external control mechanisms and enable midwives to carve out a space within which they can assert a degree of control over their work. Although a fatalistic 'there's nothing I can do about it' response may be evoked, midwives do not simply acquiesce to the external constraints that impinge upon their practice. They are active agents who utilize a variety of tactics and strategies. These enable individuals to assert their own power as the working day unfolds.

Not only is peer surveillance and regulation of clinical practice realized at times of overt information exchange, such as handover or report time in the ward office, but supervisory relationships are ongoing throughout the working day; before and after a work shift for example, when staff meet together in changing areas, or during meal and coffee breaks, or during administrative or house-keeping procedures. In order to explore the ways in which these invisible supervisory processes are worked out in practice—how midwives manage to contradict both formal and informal controls over their work—I would like to reconsider the use of the concept of 'normality' in childbirth. For although midwives are entitled to 'diagnose pregnancies and monitor normal pregnancies; to carry out examinations necessary for the monitoring of the development of normal pregnancies' (Article 4:2 of the European Community Midwives Directive), the definition of normality throughout the whole of the childbearing process is illusive. The influence that midwives and childbearing women have over the interpretation of normality is limited. Control over normality lies firmly in the hands of the medical profession. Yet midwives are imbued during their training with an expectation of responsible professional practice. This expectation is reinforced by the professional press, which, particularly since the 1979 Nurses, Midwives and Health Visitors Act drew midwifery into the centre of the nursing fold, has been vociferous in its assertion of the midwife's claim to specialist status. Fears aroused by the clinical regrading review (Cleminson Report, 1988) have also highlighted the profession's concern to demonstrate a tangible difference between the responsibilities of the midwife and those of the nurse (RCM, 1987). In a recent editorial entitled 'A midwife is a midwife is a midwife', the profession was assured that 'Midwives are, by virtue of their training, practitioners in their own right in cases of normal midwifery; i.e. for approximately 80% of the national client group' and 'midwives are empowered by statute to confirm pregnancy and undertake delivery and postnatal care without reference to a medical practitioner, provided everything progresses normally. Nurses are not in a position to exercise this type of autonomy. Midwives do not function under the direction of medical personnel. We simply refer clients to them when we identify a deviation from the normal' (MIDIRS, 1989). This stands in stark contrast to a statement issued by the Royal College of Obstetricians and Gynaecologists in 1983 in which the RCOG stated that 'The Royal College of Obstetricians cannot accept that within either the specialist maternity unit or the general practitioner unit the midwife is "responsible" for the management of all normal deliveries. Ultimate responsibility must rest with the consultants within the unit or with the general practitioner under whose care the patient is booked' (RCOG, 1983).

Control over the definition of normality, and particularly the imposition of the powerful concept of retrospective normality (the assertion that the childbearing process can only really be said to be normal in hindsight), allows representatives of the medical profession considerable room to manoeuvre within each clinical practice setting. Even when the closely guarded and seldom used label 'normal' is tentatively applied to a woman, the midwife practising in a hospital finds herself hedged in by policies and regimens, by conflicting medical truths. The opportunities that she has to apply her professional knowledge and to make decisions based upon that knowledge, even to be 'with woman' (2), are often prescribed for her. Although community midwives work under looser constraints, the pattern of clinic attendance is still usually determined by the medical profession. Whether or not the general practitioner plays an active, participatory role, he casts an ever-present shadow over proceedings. For even with the recent liberalization of antenatal clinic attendance regimens and the introduction of midwives' clinics, the midwife's access to pregnant women is controlled, to a large extent, by medical policies and procedures. The authority of the medical profession has an insidious influence over the practice of midwifery. In a busy antenatal clinic a midwife excused the long wait endured by the woman that she had examined.

If they come to the hospital clinic then they should be seen by the doctor . . . after all it's what the patient expects. It's what they come for (3).

But midwives do manage to veto medical control. Robinson *et al.* (1983)

note that 'opportunities for hospital midwives to take responsibility for complete antenatal assessments arose when medical staff referred women to midwives' clinics, when medical staff had to be absent from the clinic or when the clinic was too large for all of them to be examined by the doctor'. Midwives are therefore able to set aside the necessity for medical supervision as is evident in the following exchange that took place during a busy antenatal clinic session.

> **Midwife A**:   They're so slow. We're getting behind with the clinic, we'll never get finished.

> She turned to midwife B who was waiting outside a cubicle for a doctor to examine 'her' patient.

> **Midwife A**:   Is your woman alright? If you're happy with her just send her home.
> **Midwife B**:   Yes she's fine; I'll tell her to go then.

In intranatal care, the external constraints upon the midwife's work are widely acknowledged (Garcia *et al.*, 1985). Robinson *et al.* (1983) note that 'women in normal labour are cared for by a midwife and [are] not examined by a doctor unless the midwife asks him/her to do so' but, at the same time, 'a substantial proportion of these midwives worked in units in which certain decisions basic to the management of normal labour (for example, when to carry out vaginal examinations and at what point in labour to rupture membranes) are not made by the midwife managing the case, but are made by a doctor or are determined by unit policy'. Policies may be very specific, severely curtailing the individual's freedom to determine the care she gives to a labouring woman. Yet these constraints can be circumvented by midwives, as is evident in the following exchange which took place in a consultant unit's delivery suite. A student midwife came out of one of the labour rooms. She was taking care of a woman in her first pregnancy who was well advanced in labour. She moved to the midwives' station where the experienced staff midwife, with whom she had been allocated to work, was standing chatting to two midwifery sisters.

> **Student midwife**:   I think she might be fully [i.e. in the second stage of labour]. The epidural's wearing off and she's starting to feel some pressure. Do you want to come and have a look? Shall I get a VE trolley?
> **Midwife**:   She's not distressed is she?
> **Student midwife**:   No.
> **Midwife**:   And she's not pushing?
> **Student midwife**:   No, she's fine.

**Midwife**: Good, in that case we'll leave her for a bit. Let's go and get her sitting up and we'll see if the head will come down a bit.
**Student midwife**: So you don't want to VE her?
**Midwife**: If we can't see anything in half an hour or so, then we'll examine her . . . there's no urgency . . . if everything's fine there's no point in VE-ing her, we don't want to give them an excuse for 'helping her along'.

In choosing *not* to examine the labouring woman, the midwife is employing a strategy that enables her to maintain control; she is denying (or at least delaying) the doctors' opportunity to categorize the labour as abnormal, and therefore their opportunity to take over clinical responsibility.

During interactions between practitioners, individuals construct and exchange verbal pictures which serve to map out and reinforce the midwife's legitimate occupational space and to emphasize the special abilities attributable to members of the profession while denigrating the contribution of other 'knowledgeable doers'. In the process of 'story telling', midwives are able to construct a rational, caring depiction of midwifery and to contrast this with a non-rational, inhumane representation of other occupational groups: the 'bogey man' is characterized, categorized and coped with. Such discourse contributes to the development and maintenance of a coherent occupational identity and promotes group cohesiveness within each work setting.

The following exchange took place as the night staff handed over to day staff in a hospital maternity ward.

**Night midwife**: Mrs X was palpated as cephalic by the midwife last night, but the houseman made her a breech, so there you are! I'd rather believe the midwife any day, she's a lot more *au fait* with palpations than any houseman.

She looked to the day staff for response; there was a general nodding of heads.

**Day midwife**: And that goes for VEs too . . . they go along to assess a cervix, think of a number and write it down. It doesn't matter if the cervix is shut tight or fully dilated, they'll write down 1 to 2 centimetres anyway.

Everyone laughed: The night midwife moved on to discuss the next patient.

The following illustration was recorded as a number of midwives were drinking coffee after the conclusion of an antenatal clinic session. The bogey man is clearly of the species 'obstetrician'.

**Midwife A**:   Did you hear that woman screaming?

**Midwife B**:   I should think that everyone in the clinic heard. What on earth was going on?

**Midwife A**:   It was a postnatal. I felt awful. She's waited ages especially to see Dr A. I got the K.Y. ready for him to take a smear, but he says 'I'm gentle enough, I don't need lubrication' so then he jams in the speculum and the woman nearly shot off the end of the couch.

**Midwife C**: Ugh!

**Midwife A**:   It was awful. The poor woman did scream. Honestly, I wouldn't dream of doing that.

**Midwife B**:   When you think about how careful you are to be gentle, and to explain everything, even to an antenatal, but with a postnatal . . .

**Midwife C**:   I wouldn't choose to be treated by Dr A.

**Midwife A**:   How often does he do a smear! He's out of practice but of course they [the patients] don't know that. They think the higher up they are the better they are.

So far in this discussion I have paid scant attention to the influence that childbearing women may exert over the work of the midwife. Clearly, the childbearing woman is not merely a neutral object of work. Indeed, her active participation in the provision of maternity care may also constitute an effective source of informal control over clinical midwifery practice. At a first glance the way in which midwives interact with childbearing women appears to be inexplicably contradictory. Midwives may be supportive of childbearing women, recognizing their relative lack of power in contemporary health care, and allying the interest of the two groups of women to provide a united stand against obstetricians, as evidenced in the following conversation. This discussion took place during an afternoon handover report. A woman nearing the end of a twin pregnancy had been admitted to the ward that morning.

**Sister**:   They've left it late to bring her in.

**Staff midwife**:   She's refused a couple of times, only this time she felt he [the consultant] was getting a bit funny about it. She feels they're taking over her pregnancy from her.

**Sister**:   It's difficult to argue against them.

**Staff midwife**:   Why should she have to come in if she doesn't want to? It doesn't do her any good. She'll just get het up here and with the traffic noise she can rest much better at home.

**Sister**:   It doesn't make sense. I'll go and see how she's feeling.

The report moved on to the next patient.

The characterization of a professional practitioner that is embodied in the Code of Professional Conduct that binds all midwives (as well as nurses and health visitors) would lead us to expect to see evidence of this type of advocatory relationship between midwives and childbearing women. 'Each registered nurse, midwife and health visitor shall act at all times in such a manner as to justify public trust and confidence, to uphold and enhance the good standing and reputation of the profession, to serve the interests of society, and above all to safeguard the interests of individual patients and clients' (UKCC, 1984).

But patient advocacy and client-centred control can only go so far before it threatens to undermine the legitimacy of the midwife's role in maternity care. Midwives *do* learn to control women in a variety of ways. Informal midwifery relationships serve to keep patients or clients in their place, belying the woman's right to assert her power and legitimizing the midwife's authority as mediator between childbearing women and agents of the medical profession. The conversation noted below took place during an antenatal clinic session. The clinic procedures demand that a woman notifies her presence to the reception staff and then waits to be processed. Midwife A had collected a new patient's notes from the reception area, but had been unable to locate the woman.

Midwife A leant on a desk which guards the entrance to the clinic area. Midwife B was filling out forms. They were physically separated from the patient's waiting area by double swing doors.

**Midwife A**:  I've called this woman's name three times. I don't know where they get to.

**Midwife B**:  I know. Last week I had to call one woman I don't know how many times. I kept going back to her. She never turned up. I 'phoned her afterwards 'cos she was supposed to be having her PKU done. She said she was told to come in for a scan so she came in, had her scan then assumed she was done and went home. She never told anyone. No-one checked her over. I had to get her back the next day.

**Midwife A**:  I wouldn't be surprised at anything they do. Perhaps they think we can check them by remote control—over the phone even. I wonder what the odds are for my woman still being here. They'll have told her to come to clinic to book in so she's probably been to report to reception and now she's gone home! I'll have another go!

The women are portrayed as being feckless and incapable of understanding organizational procedures. The 'problem' is articulated in a way that incorporates a prescription for its solution. (See Moore, 1974, for discussion of this strategy.) Midwives are therefore able to perceive midwifery control as a justifiable, rational response, as the midwives in a hospital maternity ward demonstrate.

A pregnant woman presented herself at the door of the ward office. Three members of staff (two staff midwives and one student midwife) were sitting chatting in the office. They had not been notified of the woman's admission. The woman introduced herself.

**Mrs M.**:   They told me to come in.
**Staff Midwife**:   What did they tell you to come in for?
**Mrs M.**:   I don't know.
**Staff Midwife**:   Didn't you ask?

The staff midwife grunted, took the woman's antenatal clinic appointment card and led her to any empty bed in the ward before returning to the office.

**Staff Midwife**:   I can't understand why these women just do as they're told. You'd think they'd be just a little bit curious to know why they're being admitted.

[She then pulled an idiotic face and, imitating the woman, continued . . .]

'I don't know why I'm here'.
**Student Midwife**:   That's *why* they come in.

I do not mean to cast the midwife as the Machiavelli of maternity care, nor to infer that these are invidious and devious individuals. Rather, the contradictory relationships between midwives and childbearing women can be interpreted as manifestations of the relative powerlessness of midwives in contemporary health care. As they strive to confound outside influences upon midwifery, midwives have a limited range of strategies open to them and the manipulation of social relationships is one available option which the individual optimizes in order to gain a degree of control over her work.

The counter-culture that may develop within each practice setting can prove to be an extremely effective foil against the constraints experienced during the working day. But the development of effective supervisory relationships cannot be assumed. Informal processes of practice supervision may indeed not develop at all. For this unofficial supervision of midwifery work exists only as part of a fragile, dynamic culture which is contingent upon the time, the place and the individual midwives whose interactions maintain and reinforce the fluid web of relationships within the specific work setting. Yet where there is a degree of stability and continuity of staff, countercultures do develop which enable the establishment of invisible midwifery hierarchies that are separate from and which may even contradict formal position. Individuals utilize some ability or characteristic to accrue status and authority. They may have specialist practical skills, they may have developed a particular proficiency in the manipulation of administrative procedures and rules, or they may be characters or jokers, adept at social interaction. These are the midwives whose opinions are sought by their peers, whose actions are watched, and whose contribution to midwifery in their particular work setting cannot be expressed solely in terms of official rank.

The prestige that midwives in the informal hierarchy accumulate may be translated into real power when they are able to veto external control, as when, for example, individuals are able to influence the allocation of work areas. While systems of internal staff rotation between areas of antenatal, intranatal and postnatal care are now commonplace, the assignment of midwives to different areas of clinical practice after qualification is usually determined according to managerial imperative. Nevertheless, there is often a small number of individuals who manage to spend a disproportionate amount of time working in the higher status area of intranatal care while, perhaps, avoiding what is often a controversial rotation into the Special Care Baby Unit.

The informal midwifery hierarchy is also reflected in the distribution of work tasks. Activities that are considered to be peripheral to midwifery, or outside of the core of legitimate midwifery work as it is perceived in each practice setting, are most easily avoided by those midwives who have achieved an unofficial but very real standing among their peers. This is particularly true of housekeeping tasks such as damp-dusting, bed making and cleaning, and the storage of linen. The following conversation between staff in a hospital maternity ward illustrates just this:

Three staff midwives and a student midwife were sitting in the ward office in the late afternoon.

**Staff Midwife A**: I hate it when it's quiet like this, it makes the day drag.

**Staff Midwife B**: I know, the less you do the harder it is to motivate yourself.

**Staff Midwife A**: I hope the lates get back from tea in good time then we can all go home. If you lot go and put the linen away, I'll make us all a coffee. We should just have time before they get back.

**Staff Midwife C**: Isn't there an auxiliary on tonight?

**Staff Midwife A**: Afraid not . . . It'll not take long.

Staff Midwife A remained seated while the other two staff midwives and the student midwife rose and left the office.

The assertion that 'a midwife is a midwife is a midwife' (MIDIRS, 1989) clearly needs to be qualified. A very real though fragile status hierarchy is continuously produced and reproduced through the ongoing interactions of individuals and this heterogeneity among practitioners also has important implications for the process of information exchange within the workplace. Outsiders, including representatives of the medical profession, agents of management and the supervisor of midwives, are excluded from the casual conversations that take place between peers in the course of the working day.

Inter-group communication underpins the development of cultural norms and is an essential element of the assimilation of new practitioners as they enter the specific work setting. Individuals entering from other practice areas learn what is preferred, tolerated and frowned upon. The group disabuses the individual of practices that cannot be accommodated into the cultural milieux. But this is a two-way process. The individual may offer practices, attitudes or moralities for consideration by the peer group. This conversation between two midwives occurred while they were making a bed in a hospital maternity ward.

**Midwife**:　Mrs I's for Prostin tonight and induction tomorrow.
**New midwife**:　She had Prostin last night, didn't she?
**Midwife**:　Yes, poor thing. Let's hope they get her going this time.
**New midwife**:　Who gives the Prostin here?
**Midwife**:　Well, the doctor has to write it up but we can give it . . . tho' it depends who's on. If it's busy the doctors can do it. If they want it done at an awkward time then it's up to them to give it.
**New midwife**:　We hardly ever used it where I worked.
**Midwife**:　Why was that?
**New midwife**:　Only one consultant liked it . . . the others used a foleys catheter.
**Midwife**:　Oh I've heard of that but I've never seen it used. Is it any good?
[. . . the conversation continued in this vein.]

To some it may appear that the ways in which midwives define and direct their practice are so obvious that it is barely worth the effort of describing them. Certainly, supervision in midwifery has been conspicuous in the professional press largely by its absence, which is perhaps surprising, considering midwifery's long tradition of formal supervision.

From the rules, regulations and codes that govern midwives we get a definite, hard and fast picture of the midwife's role and responsibilities. Yet for the majority of midwives, informal supervision is an integral part of their daily experience of work. When *these* supervisory relationships break down, or when a problem cannot be dealt with within a particular practice setting—and midwifery clashes with the outside world, the medical profession (as opposed to an individual representative), or the public (as opposed to an individual woman or her family)—then formal supervision comes into its own. But if we fail to recognize the very real influence of the unofficial supervisory relationships that are an integral part of the culture of midwifery then an understanding of clinical midwifery practice will be denied to us.

However, one final (perhaps self-evident) point remains to be made. Any practitioner who is involved in community-based work or who works independently will recognize that this chapter is strongly biased towards the consideration of hospital midwifery. The fact that the overwhelming majority of contemporary midwives do work as employees within a bureaucratic organizational structure may, to some extent, excuse this partisan approach, but the virtual exclusion of community midwifery and independent practice from this analysis is a serious omission. All midwives are subject to the same statutory supervisory structure, and although Cronk and Flint (1989) treat the issue of formal supervision of community midwifery as non-problematic, the ways in which midwives working outside of an institutional context oversee and control their own clinical practice remain obscure.

## NOTES

1. For simplicity, midwives are referred to in the female gender throughout.
2. 'Midwife' is derived from the Old English 'mid' (with) + 'wif' (woman).
3. The illustrative case material contained in the text was obtained during a participant–observation study in a hospital maternity unit.

## REFERENCES

Cleminson Report (1988) Review Body for Nursing Staff, Midwives, Health Visitors and Professions Allied to Medicine. Fifth Report on Nursing Staff, Midwives and Health Visitors. Chairman Sir James Cleminson, CM 360, HMSO.

Cronk, M. and Flint, C. (1989) *Community Midwifery. A practical guide.* Heinemann, London.

Flint, C. (1987) Midwives' judgement, *Nursing Times*, 10 March, **83**(9), 39.

Garcia, J., Garforth, S. and Ayers, S. (1985) Midwives Confined? Labour Ward Policies and Routines. Research and the Midwife. Conference Proceedings.

Hughes, D. and Parker, O. (1987) Midwives, or Obstetricians' Disciples? *Nursing Times*, 18 Feb., **83**(6), 58.

Isherwood, K. (1988) Friend or watchdog? *Nursing Times*, 15 June, **84**(24), 65.

MIDIRS (Midwives Information and Resource Service) (1987) Interview with Mary Cronk (conducted by Jilly Rosser). MIDIRS Information Pack 4, April.

MIDIRS (Midwives Information and Resource Service) (1989) Editorial. A midwife is a midwife is a midwife. MIDIRS Information Pack No 10.

Moore, M. (1974) Demonstrating the rationality of an occupation: The depiction of their occupation by 'Progressive Clergymen'. *Sociology*, **8** (Jan.), 111–123.

*Nursing Times* (1987) 'News', Isle of Wight Midwife at Centre of Row, *Nursing Times*, 14 Jan., **83**(2), 7.

RCM (Royal College of Midwives) (1987) Evidence to the Review Body for Nursing Staff, Midwives, Health Visitors and Professions Allied to Medicine for 1987. Published Nov. 1986. Reprinted as a supplement. *Midwives Chronicle and Nursing Notes*, Jan., **100**(1), 188.

RCOG (Royal College of Obstetricians and Gynaecologists) (1983) RCOG Response to the Joint Statement on Birth and the Post-Natal Period, issued by the Health Visitors Association and the Royal College of Midwives Statement on Birth and the Post-Natal Period, RCOG, September.

Robinson, S., Golden, J. and Bradley, S. (1983) A Study of the Role and Responsibilities of the Midwife. Nursing Education Research Unit. Chelsea College. University of London.

UKCC (United Kingdom Central Council for Nursing, Midwifery and Health Visiting) (1984) Code of Professional Practice for the Nurse, Midwife and Health Visitor, 2nd edition, November. UKCC, 23 Portland Place, London.

UKCC (United Kingdom Central Council for Nursing, Midwifery and Health Visiting) (1986a) A Midwife's Code of Practice, for Midwives Practising in the United Kingdom, 1st edition, May, UKCC.

UKCC (United Kingdom Central Council for Nursing, Midwifery and Health Visiting) (1986b) Handbook of Midwives Rules, May, UKCC.

Walker, M. (1988) What is a 'practising midwife'? Letter to the Editor. *Midwife, Health Visitor and Community Nurse*, April, **25**(4), 140.

Warren, C. (1988) Scared to be midwives? *Association of Radical Midwives Magazine*, Sept., 13–14.

# CHAPTER EIGHT

# General/adult nursing

## *Jane Merchant*

## THE NATURE OF GENERAL/ADULT NURSING

That part of nursing that has been traditionally known as 'general/adult nursing' represents a very broad span of activities. In a general medical ward, for example, it is possible to find cardiology, nephrology, neurology and numerous other medically determined specialties. In surgical wards there is a similar tendency towards specialization. In addition, the kind of acute hospital-based nursing we label as 'general' also includes high technology units and accident and emergency departments. The majority of nurses working in these areas hold general registration (RGN) or enrolment (EN(G)), now referred to as first and second level registration. Some may also hold an appropriate post-basic qualification; the work force includes nurses in training and health care assistants whose role is to assist nurses.

## THE ENVIRONMENT

There have been significant organizational changes in general hospitals in the past 20 years. In particular, the turnover of patients has increased dramatically and because of early discharge policies and advances in medicine and surgery the majority of hospital in-patients either require a great deal of nursing care, or stay so briefly that relationships with nursing staff are transitory. In addition the care of patients often has a high technical component so that cardiac monitors, intravenous pumps and central venous lines are now commonplace, not only in areas defined as high technology, but in general wards. The changing pace and nature of nursing clearly has implications for 'mentors', supervisors and those they work with and supervise.

## TRADITIONAL RELATIONSHIPS IN GENERAL NURSING

The traditional apprenticeship model of nurse training has been built on a belief that practical, on-the-job experience is an ideal way to 'learn' nursing.

Providing trained nurses to ensure supervision of untrained staff and those in training was a crucial part of the Nightingale reforms in the latter half of the 19th century (Abel-Smith, 1960) and, in spite of the many changes that have taken place in the delivery of nursing and in nurse education, there is an underlying assumption in British nursing that charge nurses and sisters teach, and therefore that students learn as they work (Fretwell, 1980). The major changes heralded by Project 2000 have raised this debate to a new level and there is evidence that new and innovative approaches to student teaching will emerge for students whose commitment to rostered service has been dramatically reduced.

Although there have been many changes in title, and various reorganizations of the management of hospitals, a largely hierarchical system still persists. Resulting relationships from this system have been described by Katz and Kahn (1966) as occurring in pairs, that is, supervisor and subordinate(s). Each individual or group in the structure has a supervisor, except the head or director. Except those at the very bottom of the hierarchy, each will also have subordinates. The resulting structure stipulates the span of control of each supervisor and might be viewed as a set of power relationships. While this description might be fitted to nursing management structures, it is often difficult to decide which roles are supervisory and what a 'span of control' might be. The nursing officer role was a particularly good example of this. Many nursing officers found it difficult to define their role and authority, particularly in relation to the ward sister and this caused problems in day-to-day management. Those Nursing Officers who had most success in developing their role worked in specialist units such as intensive care, or managed units with wards of only one specialty in which they themselves had relevant expertise and therefore maintained a credibility with clinical staff (Jones, 1982).

Many hospitals are now trying to address this problem by implementing clinically orientated roles such as that of Senior Clinical Sister. This ensures that those in supervisory middle management roles have the relevant clinical knowledge and experience for their post.

The situation has been complicated by the introduction of a system of general management, a system in which some nurses now find themselves managerially accountable to a general manager, and professionally accountable to a senior nurse. Student nurses have also traditionally received supervision from both teaching and clinical staff. Such divisions of responsibility for supervision can cause friction in relationships and problems for the supervisee if expectations of supervisors differ. There are already reported cases where professional expectations (determined by the UKCC Code of Professional Conduct for nurses) might be at odds with the employer's expectations and demands.

## MENTORS AND MENTORSHIP IN ADULT/GENERAL NURSING

Although Hagerty (1986) has noted the 'definition quagmire' around the role of mentor, Kramer (1972) has proposed that a mentor is a nurse who manages to blend value systems from education programmes and the workplace and in this way defuses possible conflicts that may arise between the two.

Puetz (1985) suggests various functions for mentors including those of teacher, sponsor, host, exemplar and counsellor. Various reports of introducing mentorship schemes can be found in the literature. Raichura and Riley (1985) reported the introduction of 'nurse preceptors' in a ward for elderly people and recommend nurses with a strong clinical base and up-to-date knowledge for this role. Northcott (1989) has described the system as used in one college of nursing where mentors are expected to be familiar with the curriculum and the expected competencies to be achieved during the placement of students. Clinical mentors are selected and prepared by specifically designed programmes. Laurent (1988) describes the system introduced in Oxford where students have an identified tutor throughout their course and staff nurse 'mentors' are identified for each clinical experience in general/adult wards.

This growing literature supports the case that mentorship is receiving considerable attention in general/adult nursing.

## DEFINING SUPERVISION

It is difficult to find a definition of supervision in nursing literature and those available tend to concentrate on a definition which considers the management aspects. Yura *et al.* (1981) suggest that supervision occurs at the level of management where activities are operationalized, having been delegated down from other levels. It is used to ensure that work is carried out and means 'to oversee, to inspect or to peruse'. Kron (1981) suggests that supervision is difficult to define but that it should be democratic rather than autocratic and that it is easier to list the qualities of a good supervisor than to say what supervision is. Beyers and Philips (1979) discuss the concepts of 'general' and 'close' supervision but believe that individual supervisors should choose a style which suits themselves and their area of work, and that nurses of differing personalities will choose to work in different units.

The teaching aspect of supervision, which is so much part of the British nurse education system, is not really accounted for in these essentially managerial definitions of supervision, although Kron (1981) does suggest that supervision involves using teaching skills to help the worker. However, it is the teaching aspect of supervision which probably causes the most concern to general nurses. How much and what type of supervision should be given to untrained staff and students is a major concern both in order to facilitate patient care and to provide learning opportunities for students. Ensuring that students receive supervised practice in order that they learn particular procedures has traditionally been viewed as an important part of their experience but the relationship between giving supervision and teaching has not been thoroughly examined.

## THE ROLE OF THE SUPERVISOR

In view of the great changes that have occurred in general nursing, it appears self-evident that accompanying changes should have been made in supervisory relationships. The General Nursing Council, and more recently the United Kingdom Central Council for Nursing, Midwifery and Health Visiting (UKCC), have continued to assume that supervision of students will be carried out during clinical allocations. They have not, however, defined supervision but have tended to concentrate on the ratio of trained staff to learners in clinical areas. This approach seems to assume that all qualified nurses are adequately prepared for teaching, understand the relationship between teaching and supervision and are willing to take on the supervisory role.

Argyle (1979) describes supervision as a situation in which one person has to ensure that work is carried out properly. The supervisor does not do the work himself but inspects, supervises the procedure or assists with the work. Since the relationship between supervisor and worker is so close, the social skills of the supervisor may affect job satisfaction, staff turnover and absenteeism. In Argyle's view, the supervisor's job may be difficult for several reasons:

1. the technological setting;
2. because of vulnerability to pressures from both management and workers;
3. because he usually supervises a group and must be seen to treat each individual fairly, despite differences in age, personality and skills.

For nurses supervising staff in busy general wards, these difficulties will also occur. In this case, the supervision of work concerns the care of those who are very ill and the question of what work to delegate and how much supervision to give is a potential cause of stress especially for newly qualified staff nurses (Walker, 1986). Even an experienced ward sister is vulnerable to pressures which make the role difficult, for example, from her own staff, the needs of patients and relatives, the medical staff and the hospital administration (Mauksch, 1966). In addition, the ward sister usually works in a situation where up to 50% of her staff are untrained or in training, she has little or no power over the selection and de-selection of staff, and there are frequent changes of personnel, especially students (Pembrey, 1980). Although everyone who works in a general nursing setting may have difficulties in their work and relationships because of the structure and environment, the three groups who are particularly affected are charge nurses or ward sisters, newly qualified staff nurses and students and these groups will be discussed in more detail in the remainder of this chapter.

### THE CHARGE NURSE/WARD SISTER

The charge nurse/ward sister is the key person in the ward, that is, the coordinator of all activities and communications. She is responsible for the standard of nursing care and for the organization of all work that is carried out in the ward, including the orientation of new staff and teaching of students (Pembrey, 1980). According to some literature on managing organizations, the charge nurse/ward sister occupies a typical supervisory position, that is, she is responsible for and must achieve work through others. In a creative analysis, Pembrey (1980) has used an approach based on systems theory and argued that the hospital ward has changed over the years from a comparatively closed to an open system. This suggests that a complex web of influences are at play in any ward environment and likely to be beyond the control of any single person.

The accessibility and openness of wards and the resulting interruptions in the charge nurse/ward sister's work have frequently been cited as a reason why they may fail to fulfil their role (Lelean, 1973). Given the complexity of their role and the lack of formal preparation, it is perhaps not surprising that research suggests that students do not always receive the amount of supervision and teaching that might be considered desirable (Farnish, 1982; Merchant, 1982).

Research into the ward learning environment confirms that it is the charge nurse/ward sister who is the major influence here too (Orton, 1981; Ogier, 1982). Unfortunately, the situation where students are viewed as workers often leads to their being used to undertake the most routine work on the ward. This is not conducive to learning and is likely to inhibit the spirit of enquiry (Fretwell, 1980). It is now usual for charge nurses/ward sisters to learn some teaching and assessment skills through the English National Board 998 Course. This does not, however, address itself to the complex problem of how a ward sister manages a ward in order to facilitate a high standard of patient care whilst ensuring that students' learning objectives are met.

There has been a tendency to define some nursing work as 'basic' and to assume that those in training can safely carry out such work. This has resulted in a large proportion of nursing care being carried out by untrained staff and such supervision as has occurred has been concentrated on the so-called 'technical' tasks (e.g. caring for intravenous infusions; giving drugs). This has tended to perpetuate a hierarchy of tasks (Merchant, 1985) and prevents students from obtaining a holistic view of patient care. The system of organizing nursing care, usually called task allocation, requires that the sister, or nurse in charge, plans the care for all patients. This is then broken down into tasks and each nurses is assigned a task or group of tasks. This results in junior students undertaking baths and other tasks associated with patients' personal hygiene. Senior students and trained nurses would be involved in dressing wounds and giving drugs (Merchant, 1985). Students, therefore, tend to be viewed as workers competent to undertake specific tasks according to their stage in training (Burkey, 1984), and the system reinforces the idea that the work is more important than the individual patient (Fretwell, 1980).

If this situation is to change it is necessary for the management of wards to be geared towards a model which allows student nurses to observe the professional practice of nursing. At present qualified nurses, especially sisters, spend a very small proportion of their working day involved in direct patient care. This may result in students viewing senior ward staff as office managers. The role model is known to be a strong influence on future practice (Pembrey, 1980) but the concept is complex and there is some evidence to suggest that poor practice is sometimes influential (Merchant, 1982; Walker, 1986). The practice of team or primary nursing by effectively prepared staff can, however, maximize the opportunities for students to observe qualified nurses involved in all aspects of patient care.

Team nursing is the allocation of a small group of nurses (a team) to a group of patients for whose care they are responsible throughout their stay in hospital. A registered nurse is the team leader who must exercise leadership and management skills in order to promote optimum standards of nursing care (Waters, 1985). The ward sister may function as a team leader or may be freed to act as a consultant and/or teacher. Students can be allocated to a particular team, under the guidance of the team leader, during their allocation to the ward. Depending upon their level of experience, they will work alongside other members of the team or take responsibility for a particular patient or patients. The team leader, however, remains accountable for the standard of care. In this way, students can be given responsibility according to their experience and gain confidence in a supportive environment. Team nursing requires commitment from all ward staff and will fail if nurses do not understand the concept and use the team structure to allocate tasks on a hierarchical basis.

Primary nursing is the system where a specific registered nurse is responsible for a particular group of patients throughout their stay in hospital (Lee, 1979). In particular, this nurse carries out the assessment and care planning for each patient although she/he may not give all the care. Each primary nurse has several patients to care for (the actual number depending upon the dependency of the patients) and will have one or more associate nurses who will help to care for these patients. In Great Britain the associate nurse is usually a newly registered or an enrolled nurse. The primary nurse is accountable for the patients' care at all times. Students may be allocated to the care of a particular primary nurse while on the ward. The student will work alongside the primary nurse or may function as an associate nurse, with some support if she/he is nearing completion of training. This method offers the student a role model who is actively involved in clinical practice. It also provides a supportive environment which can serve to prepare a student for the responsibilities which come with registration. The ward sister may function as a primary nurse or may choose the role of ward coordinator and be free to function as advisor and teacher to the benefit of all staff.

Ward sisters who have functioned in a traditional manner may find it difficult to adapt to these different methods of ward organization. In particular, they may be very uncomfortable if they feel less in 'control' of a busy, acute ward (Binnie, 1989). However, the benefits that accrue to all the staff in having the most experienced nurse on the ward freed to act either as a primary nurse, or to act as a clinical consultant, are enormous.

The charge nurse/ward sister is a key to the success of any change in organizational style. It is important, therefore, that sisters are given the management support and continued education required to implement changes that would be beneficial to all staff.

## THE NEWLY REGISTERED NURSE

In both team and primary nursing systems the accountability for patient care falls to registered nurses, usually of staff nurse grade. There is already evidence to suggest that newly registered nurses find their transition from the student role very stressful (Lathlean, 1987; Walker, 1986). This is a group of staff for whom personal supervision and support suddenly ceases with the acquisition of a professional qualification. Overnight they are expected to function as qualified nurses and to teach and supervise others. In fact, delegation and supervision of work are areas they may experience difficulty with. Having delegated work they may worry about how well it is being done; they find it hard to trust students to perform at the right standard and as a consequence often check up on staff frequently. At the same time, their relationship with other staff has changed and they may worry about being viewed as 'bossy' or as not doing a fair share of the work. This can conflict with the need to maintain the ward routine and get work done by the end of a shift, particularly if this appears to be part of the ward sister's expectations of her staff nurses (Walker, 1986).

Recent evidence suggests that it is usual for staff nurses to be expected to manage wards immediately they qualify; however, in at least one study ward sisters expressed reservations about whether newly qualified staff nurses had the skills to function as team leaders (Merchant, 1982). Apart from clinical knowledge, leadership and management skills are required to function as a team leader or primary nurse. Orientation to the new role and support in the clinical area are important and can form part of a post-registration professional development course. Such courses are in existence in some Health Authorities and provide role-based training for all newly registered nurses (Lathlean, 1987). In North America a preceptorship system is sometimes used to support and guide the neophyte staff nurse (Benner, 1982). Each newly qualified nurse is provided with a preceptor (or mentor) to guide and support and, therefore, ensure that individuals are fully orientated to their new role. Where team or primary nursing have been implemented, a staff nurse could also function as a deputy team leader or associate nurse and receive the same kind of attention.

Where no development course or preceptorship system is available, it is important that the ward sister takes responsibility for supporting newly qualified nurses and especially for offering feedback on how the nurse is adapting to the new role. In some instances, it might be possible for the continuing education department to provide a mentor who could give support in the clinical situation. If this is not possible, a member of staff could be made available to support staff in their initial months of transition. Whatever the system adopted, it is important that this group of staff who have a key influence on standards of patient care and who are involved in the teaching of students receive adequate support and supervision themselves. The organization of work in wards must take into consideration the prime function of providing a high standard of patient care but an important secondary function of whatever method is chosen is that it offers opportunities for the support and development of staff. If the charge nurse/ward sister is able to make the necessary adjustment in her role to facilitate team or primary nursing, she will be free in her new role to supervise more junior staff and make staff development a priority (Binnie, 1989).

## THE STUDENT

Few studies of student nurse learning focus on the question of supervision, but findings suggest that the ward environment may not be conducive to learning. Learning appears to be dependent on the atmosphere created by the ward sister and there may be observable differences between wards in the same hospital (Fretwell, 1980; Ogier, 1982). Orton (1981) described this as 'high student orientation' and 'low student orientation'.

There is agreement in the literature that the positive aspects of ward atmosphere for students are dependent upon the sister's attitude to them. Sisters who are approachable and view students as learners rather than 'pairs of hands' promote a positive learning environment while routinized work and repetitive tasks are considered to be 'the antithesis of a learning environment' (Fretwell, 1980). The way the ward is organized and the attitudes of the staff therefore may also be major factors in ensuring a suitable learning environment.

The implementation of a system of work such as team nursing which allows for support and supervision of the student (however busy the ward) is obviously important. The team organization can take into consideration the dependency of individual patients and any special knowledge and skills required to nurse them. Where such a system is not in operation, the degree of responsibility given to students and the amount of supervision exercised may need to be judged almost on an hour by hour basis as the condition of acutely ill patients changes. Organizational strategies such as team nursing, therefore, have advantages for the ward manager as well as students. Wards already practising team nursing and primary nursing will probably find it relatively easy in the future to adapt to students having supernumerary status, for example, by gradually increasing the amount of involvement the student has in the nursing team.

The preparation of qualified nurses for their teaching role is also important as their perception of what teaching entails may be coloured by their own experience as students. For example, certain tasks and procedures may be viewed as suitable vehicles for teaching, e.g. drug rounds, while other opportunities are missed. In the past there may also have been a view that certain tasks should be supervised because they were the focus of student assessments. Therefore, it may have been local policy that such items of care as wound dressings should be supervised until such time as students had passed the relevant assessment. Students themselves may have contributed to this by requesting supervision for aseptic dressing technique and the administration of drugs because they wished to 'practise' before undertaking an assessment. This has supported a view that supervision was required for certain 'technical' tasks and in some cases may have perpetuated task allocation (Merchant, 1985) which Fretwell (1980) suggested may stifle the potential of learners. Programmes of continuous assessment, changing methods of work organization and preparing qualified nurses for their teaching role are important in eradicating this sort of task hierarchy.

A change of philosophy is required to ensure that the division of nursing work into the categories 'basic' and 'technical' does not persist. It can be argued that this division is based upon a questionable idea that so-called 'basic' care is simpler to deliver. However, the acutely ill patient with severe pain who cannot wash or move himself is in need of 'basic' care but it requires skill and expertise to meet this patient's needs without causing him more distress. It is important that this care should be given by the experienced nurse not by the untrained (Pembrey, 1984). In a primary nursing setting, this is possible and the student can work alongside the primary nurse learning these skills.

Another system which can be successfully used to ensure students receive adequate supervision is mentorship. Whatever method of ward organization is used it is possible to allocate a friend or mentor to each student from among the qualified nurses on the ward. The mentor and student discuss the student's learning objectives and particular needs at the commencement of the student's allocation, and plan particular experiences to be undertaken. This might include orientation to the ward, particular clinical skills or preparation of a care study. The off duty rota is arranged so that the student and mentor work together at least once or twice a week. This system is likely to work more successfully in a team or primary nursing setting where the student and mentor can work regularly together and care for the same group of patients throughout their stay in hospital. It can also be used as a staff development tool by gradually allocating more senior students to staff nurses as they themselves gain more experience and confidence. Preparation for the mentor role is important and will include understanding of teaching and learning theories and counselling skills, and can be undertaken both by the charge nurse/ward sister and more formally through a continuing education programme.

## CONCLUSION

The answers to problems surrounding the question of supervision will not be solved only by defining more clearly what is meant by the term. Rather it is necessary to redefine organizational relationships in hospital wards by promoting a professional model of nursing. This involves developing the skills and abilities of the general nurse so that she/he can function as a team leader or primary nurse, and deliver and be accountable for a high standard of nursing care. These roles then provide opportunities for role modelling and for students to practise under supervision. The advantage of such models of practice is that they provide benefit not just for the student. In fact, the main beneficiary is the patient who should receive more individualized and holistic care.

## REFERENCES

Abel-Smith, B. (1960) *A History of the Nursing Profession*, Heinemann, London.
Argyle, M. (1979) *The Social Psychology of Work*, Pelican Books, Harmondsworth.
Benner, P. (1982) From novice to expert, *American Journal of Nursing*, **82**(3), 402–407.
Beyers, M. and Philips, C. (1979) *Nursing Management for Patient Care*, Little, Brown & Co., Boston.
Binnie, A. (1989) Primary nursing: Where to start, *Nursing Times*, **85**(24), 43–44.
Burkey, B. P. (1984) Student Nurses' Perception of Their Training, Unpublished M.Sc. Thesis, University of Manchester.
Farnish, S. (1982) 'Thrown in at the deep end', *Nursing Times*, **78**(10), 404–405.
Fretwell, J. E. (1980) Hospital ward routine – friend or foe? *Journal of Advanced Nursing*, **5**(6), 625–636.
Hagerty, B. (1986) A second look at mentors, *Nursing Outlook*, **34**, 1.
Jones, D. (1982) The role of the nursing officer. Some implications of research, *Nursing Times*, **78**(9), 376–378.
Katz, D. and Kahn, R. L. (1966) *Social Psychology of Organisations*, John Wiley and Sons, Inc., New York.

Kramer, M. (1972) The concept of modelling as a teaching strategy, *Nursing Forum*, **11**, 50–69.

Kron, T. (1981) *The Management of Patient Care*, W. B. Saunders Company, Philadelphia.

Lathlean, J. (1987) Are you prepared to be a Staff Nurse? *Nursing Times*, **83**(36), 25–27.

Laurent, C. (1988) On hand to help, *Nursing Times*, 16 Nov., **84**(46).

Lee, M. E. (1979) Towards better care: Primary nursing, *Nursing Times*, Occasional Paper, **75**(51), 133–135.

Lelean, S. R. (1973) *Ready for Report Nurse?* A study of nursing communication in hospital wards. The Study of Nursing Care Project Reports. Series 2, No. 2, London, RCN.

Mauksch, H. O. (1966) The organisational context of nursing practice, in *The Nursing Profession: 5 Sociological Essays* (Ed. F. Davis), J. Wiley and Sons, New York.

Merchant, S. J. (1982) A Study of the Role of the Ward Sister in the Management of Patient Care, Unpublished M.Sc. Thesis, University of Manchester.

Merchant, J. (1985) Organising nursing care: Why task allocation? *Nursing Practice*, **1**(2), 67–71.

Northcott, N. (1989) Mentorship in nurse education, *Nursing Standard*, 11 March, **3**(24), 24–26.

Ogier, M. E. (1982) *An Ideal Sister?* A study of the leadership style and verbal interactions of Ward Sisters with Nurse Learners in General Hospitals, RCN, London.

Orton, H. D. (1981) Ward learning climate and student nurse response, *Nursing Times*, Occasional Paper, **77**(17), 65–68.

Pembrey, S. E. M. (1980) *The Ward Sister – Key to Nursing. A Study of the Organisation of Individualised Nursing*, RCN, London.

Pembrey, S. (1984) Nursing care: Professional progress, *Journal of Advanced Nursing*, **9**(6), 539–547.

Puetz, B. E. (1985) Learn the ropes from a mentor, *Nursing Success Today*, **2**(6), 11–13.

Raichura, E. and Riley, M. (1985) Introducing nurse preceptors, *Nursing Times*, **81**, 20 Nov.

Walker, C. A. (1986) The Newly Qualified Staff Nurse's Perception of the Transition from Student to Trained Nurse, unpublished M.Sc. Thesis, University of Manchester.

Waters, K. (1985) Organising nursing care: Team nursing, *Nursing Practice*, **1**(1), 7–15.

Yura, H., Ozimek, D. and Walsh, M. B. (1981) *Nursing Leadership: Theory and Process*, Appleton-Century-Crofts, New York.

# CHAPTER NINE

# Mental handicap nursing

*Peggy Cooke*

## INTRODUCTION

Mental handicap nursing involves considerable liaison with other professionals and a multidisciplinary approach in resolving many of the problems that arise. It has bridged the distances between the multidisciplinary team, often working as partners with clients. Sharing buildings, offices and sometimes a manager common to other professionals has put mental handicap nurses in a unique position. Some difficulties relating to accountability for the community mental handicap nurse have been identified (Carr *et al.*, 1980) although on the whole this working together can and does work provided all professionals involved want it to work. The methods of supervision used in community mental handicap teams vary considerably, often depending very much on the structure of a particular team. Some methods may be less orthodox in that people from other disciplines are involved in the supervision of nurses.

Some might argue that, as qualified professionals, community mental handicap nurses with three or maybe four years' experience have the skills to do their work with minimal or no supervision and indeed must be allowed this freedom as independent practitioners. An alternative argument is that the nurse needs continuous supervision thereby ensuring that a high quality and cost-effective service is provided and that this accountability helps to provide clients with a good service and community mental handicap nurses with a future.

Supervising the clinical practice of the mental handicap nurse was and still is relatively easy in a large institutional setting. On each ward there are a number of staff ranked in order of seniority. These people have various tasks to carry out and on numerous occasions during each day/week these tasks are observed by other people both on and off the ward.

The very fact that more than one nurse is present in most situations ensures that some sort of supervision occurs at most times. In the past this supervision has been notably absent (DHSS, 1974) and in large remote psychiatric hospitals, so clearly described by Towell (1975), institutionalism, in all its damaging manifestations, has been the order of the day. In these circumstances, supervision has sought to maintain the often unhealthy status quo rather than provide quality services. Happily these situations are becoming less common and present day practices allow for relatively easy access of senior nurses or managers thus allowing problems either to be passed on for appropriate action by others or dealt with fairly quickly by the manager concerned.

As well as having a supervisory overview of a nurse's practice, the hospital environment also allows for good practice to be noted (if not rewarded) by peers or superiors. Even within this environment the practice of individual nurses has its limitations. Although nurses within hospitals are observed by others they are only rarely provided with structured supervisory sessions.

The recent wholesale moves by residents from hospital to community has resulted in the splitting up of large groups of people with a mental handicap into a much greater number of small groups. It has also resulted in many nurses working individually as autonomous practitioners. The community mental handicap nurse receives a referral and works with a family who have a handicapped member or works with a person with a mental handicap who lives alone. This freedom to work alone demands more rather than less supervision both to protect the nurse and the person with a mental handicap and/or his family.

When working in the community the mental handicap nurse is working with a vulnerable group. Carers are often at the end of their tether before they will ask for help. They perhaps have nowhere else and no-one else to go to. The problems they have are not ones that they, their relatives or neighbours can resolve by themselves and so they will turn for professional help. Service provision by community mental handicap nurses may be so new that carers have little information on, let alone experience of, services involving nurses. It is more than likely that they will have little idea what the community mental handicap nurse will be able to offer them.

Consequently, carers may accept help from nurses without knowing that alternatives may be available or equally they may believe that community mental handicap nurses cannot help them because the nurse concerned does not have the skills to meet their needs. If carers have little experience of community mental handicap nurses and what they can do, it follows they have no measure on which to base whether they are receiving a good, bad or indifferent service. This being the case there is a strong argument to monitor the services offered by the community mental handicap nurse and provide consumers with a measure of what would constitute a reasonable service.

A similar situation occurs when the person with a mental handicap, who lives independently, requires a service. That individual may have been dependent on others for many years, often not being given a choice or a say in what happens to his life. When he or she achieves a degree of independence they are often still dependent on service providers for some help. Help is particularly important when they have not been able to develop a network of contacts in their own locality. This lack of contact often compounded by a lack of opportunity to voice opinions may result in clients who will accept anything on offer. The community mental handicap nurse holds a very powerful position as gatekeeper to service provision and can, sometimes unintentionally, place their values onto the person with a mental handicap or make that person more dependent than he or she needs to be. Supervision can assist in reducing this difficulty. Once again this highlights the need for a structure of supervision within community mental handicap nursing services, ensuring a service quality within which power is placed with the right people.

Clinical supervision for mental handicap nurses is an issue that raises much discussion. Mental handicap nurses are numerically small and consequently may be managed by people from other specialist or professional backgrounds. In many areas community mental handicap nurses have worked as members of a multidisciplinary team and so may be supervised either directly or indirectly by other team members from a variety of disciplines. The nurse manager in some services may be from the mental handicap field but also may be from other areas of the nursing profession with little or no knowledge of the specialty. A recent move in some areas has seen the appointment of a team manager responsible for the community mental handicap team as a whole. This results in nurses having a manager perhaps from their own profession but equally possible their manager may be from social work or psychology, bringing with them their own professional ideologies. These recent changes in the management structure have resulted in a need for various forms of clinical supervision to enable nurses to get the support, advice and skills they need. The type of supervision provided will be very much shaped by the nurses' needs, the structure of the team and the type of management provided in that particular area.

## THE MULTIDISCIPLINARY TEAM

In a large number of community mental handicap teams a variety of professionals meet together on a regular basis—maybe weekly or fortnightly. These meetings may be referred to as multidisciplinary team meetings or core team meetings. The membership of these meetings will vary from area to area depending on how the full team has been divided up. In some areas a geographical split occurs, other areas are divided up according to the age range of the clients whilst others are defined according to the groups of people they work with, for example, resettlement teams or challenging behaviour teams. The dividing up of teams naturally results in specialisms occurring and also results in very small groups of people working together—perhaps only one of each discipline. Division of the team results in a need to rely on other, like-minded people for support and advice even if they are from another discipline.

No matter how the mental handicap team has been sub-divided, it is usual to find a variety of professionals working together in it. This will often include community mental handicap nurses and social workers, psychologists and maybe other workers like the occupational therapist, physiotherapist, speech therapist, specialist health visitor and consultant psychiatrist.

The team may meet regularly and yet offer nothing more than an information sharing forum—a team member speaks, the minute writer records, the team passes on to the next item or person on the agenda. This may be a quick and easy way of gathering information on large numbers of the client group served. It is not, however, a means of finding out if the clients needs are being met, nor is it a way of identifying if the nurse needs help or if she needs to consider an alternative approach to her work, both of which are essential to good case management. The above approach allows for those who want to contribute to do so but also allows others to give minimal or no contributions to the meeting.

An alternative approach can be and is used in some multidisciplinary team meetings which actively encourages each member's contribution. It offers a means of identifying a nurse's approach to case work and allows for discussion of alternative approaches. Input from other members of the team can help to identify areas of weakness. This type of format not only applies to nurses but to all professionals working within a team of that nature. Each group member presents a case or cases at the meeting so providing some background information, identification of the problem area(s) and the work they are doing. If more than one team member is involved with a particular client a joint presentation can be used. The individual key worker may have difficulties identifying the next step with a particular client or family—a brief brainstorming session may identify a number of approaches which could be used.

Meetings of this sort can identify particular skills of the individual and also highlight other skills within the group and sources of help if further learning has been identified. The very fact that the group contains people from different professional backgrounds means that individual case presenters have a variety of people to draw on.

Although in a strict sense this may not be considered by some to be a form of clinical supervision, it clearly offers a system of accountability to other team members and a network of support to both validate and improve upon practice. For a team of this sort to work effectively there is a need for mutual trust, honesty and openness. Equally there must be recognition of the different professional backgrounds people come from. As membership of the team is fairly fixed, relationships and knowledge of people's skills can be built on over a period of time.

It might be argued that people from a different discipline cannot supervise the clinical practice of a nurse and in some situations that may be true. However, the nature of the care needed by the person with a mental handicap is such that no one professional can be said to have all the skills or all the answers. There are many grey areas where a number of professionals may have similar skills to offer an individual or his carers. People from all disciplines have a contribution to make and each may help the other in identifying an individual's particular strengths or weaknesses.

The individual programme planning system used by many community mental handicap teams is another means whereby a team of people might supervise one another's practice. The individual programme planning system requires a group of professionals, who are working with a person with a mental handicap involving that individual and his or her carers. The intention of this meeting is to plan and coordinate the means of meeting that individual's needs. The recording of each professional's agreed contribution to meet an individual's needs and the accountability expected at the next meeting highlights the suitability of practice over a given period of time. This is a system of supervision by a variety of interested people who may or may not be nurses.

## SUPERVISION ON A ONE-TO-ONE BASIS

Supervision by a nurse manager is provided in almost all areas and may take a variety of forms depending on the working background of the manager concerned, their particular interests and other commitments. If the manager has a mental handicap background then at least she will have had some experience of working with the client group concerned, even if that experience only covers a narrow area perhaps based on in-patient care.

Regardless of the manager's background it is likely that the supervision of a nurse's case work and practice will involve not only the quality of practice but also the quantity and naturally the cost-effectiveness of the nurse's work. When considering the manager's perspective it is recognized that in today's political climate there is a need for accountability and value for money. The team manager needs a system to give an account of staff time but they must also be able to record the nurse's achievements. The use of staff time can be recorded on the forms each nurse is asked to complete on a weekly or monthly basis. Although it can be a paper pushing exercise, it is often used to decide on the budget for future years. This form at best lists a record of how many visits, meetings or programmes a community mental handicap nurse has carried out over a given period of time. As a record of the nurse's accountability it is inadequate. Other methods of supervision of a face-to-face nature must be used to ensure the quality of the nurse's clinical practice.

When measuring the quality of care, difficulties may arise because judgements are made by people about other people. If the manager likes the nurse she may think the work she does must be good. There is a need for objectivity. The use of a care plan may help the manager achieve this. If the nurse identifies needs and can prioritize them, then plans can be put into motion to achieve them. If realistic goals are set the supervisor can then see what progress has been made. By using the case note format for supervisory sessions these may then be structured. The manager may decide to go on home visits with the nurse and following that discuss her work or she may just read the case notes and discuss her observations from there.

## SUPERVISION OF THE HOME VISIT

Although observing the home visit may be a means of supervising a community mental handicap nurse's practice, it must be acknowledged that a joint visit may change the nature of the interaction between client or carer and nurse. The trust to discuss personal issues may take weeks, months or even years to build up and, therefore, the involvement of a relative stranger may result in resistance by client or carer. Parents describe this need for trust in an article by MacLachlan *et al.* (1987). They reported that 'in the early years the professional who gave the most help was the one with whom we had built up a situation of trust'. The supervisor must take guidance from the nurse regarding whether it is appropriate to visit a particular client. Supervision of the nurse must be of a positive nature, not detrimental to the working relationship with a family.

The use of the home visit as a means of supervision is helpful but it is important to foresee possible problems. It is the only accurate means of seeing how a nurse interacts with a client or carer. A visit of this nature should be carefully planned and permission from the client or carer should be obtained. This does, however, leave the supervisor in the possible position of only observing the nurse's practice when he or she has established a good working relationship. The need for supervision of the community mental handicap nurse's practice may be more necessary in homes where underlying problems exist between client/carer and nurse.

A number of alternative approaches can be used if the supervisor's presence in the client's home is felt to be inadvisable. The team meetings described earlier are one option; other possible strategies are discussed further in this chapter.

The discussion of a particular case in conjunction with a nurse's case records is a popular means of supervision. This can be useful, not only as a means of looking at a community mental handicap nurse's practice but also for looking at the recording methods used.

As a method of improving the poor recording of a good practitioner this method is useful, however, the discussion method may not highlight the problems of a poor practitioner who has good recording skills; deficits in skill can only be truly measured by observed practice. The need for a planned approach, a clear structure and succinct notes is of great importance. Preparation time needed for this may be great but keeping notes up to date is possibly less time consuming in the long run and gives a clear picture of clinical practice.

If supervision sessions are planned in advance with an informal agenda then both nurse and supervisor have a structure to follow and progress can be made. It is useful to keep some notes of the topics covered within a supervisory session and of any action agreed as this can be referred to at a later date.

## THE ROLE PLAY SITUATION

An approach which can display a nurse's practice without affecting the nurse–client relationship is the role play situation. This may only involve nurse and supervisor but can involve a number of mental handicap nurses and/or other community mental handicap team members. Individuals can then act out situations to which each member will respond. One difficulty is 'first night nerves', but if the role play situation is planned thoughtfully and with emphasis on improving the nurse's skills and providing opportunities for learning, then these nerves can be overcome. The situation can be a learning experience for all involved and need not just be a one-off activity. If, for example, the first situation is an initial visit following referral, further role play situations could reflect subsequent visits. This role play situation can also be used by the supervisor to model techniques to the nurse which he or she can use in the home.

Role play as a method of supervision need not be any more time consuming than a discussion session with the manager. A 20 minute or half-hour session is adequate to see how someone reacts and deals with a particular problem or need. Naturally, a feedback session is essential and the sooner this takes place the better, as the situation will still be fresh in the minds of all concerned. A spectator/observer is useful for feedback on specific areas of the 'actors'' performance. The feedback session allows opportunity to discuss the approach used, what alternatives could be considered, what were the good points of the interview, how the 'actors' felt in the situation and whether or not the nurse felt she had the adequate skills to deal with the situation that was presented. Any feedback can be used either within future supervisory sessions or maybe as the basis to develop staff training sessions.

## THE USE OF VIDEO EQUIPMENT

Many community mental handicap teams have access to video equipment and this has a variety of uses within supervisory sessions. The role play situation described above is one use for this equipment. The recording can be played back to support the discussion that follows. If video tapes are kept over a period of time (with the consent of all concerned) changes in the community mental handicap nurse's approach to situations can be highlighted.

Mental handicap nurses also use the camera in other situations, for example, in group sessions with clients or as a means of identifying the possible causes and responses to a particular behaviour displayed by a client. This video material can be used in supervision or peer review sessions (again with the consent of the client(s)) as a means of identifying the type of work a particular nurse is involved in. It can also be used to identify the approaches used in a particular session or as a way of enlisting the help and advice of others.

## WHO SUPERVISES THE COMMUNITY MENTAL HANDICAP NURSE?

Community mental handicap nurses are frequently supervised by their nurse managers, however, some teams recognize that managers may not have sufficient time to give adequate supervision to all staff members. Equally nurse managers may not have the specific skills that a particular member of staff is looking for. In these situations additional support may be provided by experienced community mental handicap nurses with an interest in supervision and in teaching and learning techniques. The nurses may provide this supervision on an informal, *ad hoc* basis in between the structured supervisory sessions of the manager. Alternatively a nurse's skills in this area may have been identified by their manager and are used in a structured way to help inexperienced nurses.

One-to-one supervision by a colleague (peer review) can present problems so there is a need to think clearly through any plans for its implementation. The nurse being supervised must be willing to have that supervision from someone other than their manager. There is a need for close liaison between nurse supervisor and manager to ensure that similar guidance is being given by both. Guidelines should be set so that nurse supervisors know their remit but also so that nurses being supervised know which issues to take to their nurse colleague and which to take to their manager.

The argument for a clinical nurse specialist to look at all aspects of supervision in the community mental handicap nursing field can be supported, particularly in the present climate of management restructuring. This restructuring has resulted in locality managers being drawn from district nursing or health visiting backgrounds and being directly responsible for community mental handicap nursing services. An alternative to locality managers in use in some authorities is community mental handicap team managers, from nursing but possibly from other professional backgrounds.

Balcombe (1989) highlights the need for clinical nurse specialists to have an appropriate post-basic ENB qualification, clinical teaching qualifications and some training in staff development. Many community mental handicap nurses have an appropriate ENB certificate and some of these have at least City and Guilds 730, Further Education Teachers Certificate. These nurses have the knowledge and experience to monitor their nursing colleagues and to set the standards of practice in their particular area. Many have leadership skills and are able to manage staff supervision. What they need is a reduced caseload in order to carry out this work effectively and to keep up to date with current developments.

## NURSE MEETINGS

In many community mental handicap teams nurses meet together with others from their own profession. This group may or may not include their nurse manager and the title of the group may vary accordingly—usually peer group/review meeting without the manager, or nurses' meeting/forum with the manager present.

As with the multidisciplinary team meeting the format of nurses' meetings can vary from information-giving exercises to supervision of clinical nurse practice. Although both types of meeting are important the two should not be confused.

Bullough *et al.* (1983), referring to peer review, indicate that the process is used to appraise the quality of a nurse's performance. They also indicate that it is conducted by a group of nurses actively engaged in some component of nursing practice. This group situation provides nurses with the forum that a one-to-one nurse/supervisor situation cannot provide by the very fact that nurses meet with similar practitioners. This meeting is vitally important particularly as community mental handicap nurses are so few in number and are often working in other areas of specialism or geography, so need the opportunity to share experiences, concerns, ideas and skills.

The peer review situation offers a variety of experience and expertise from a group of like-minded professionals, offering mutual support to its members.

## CONCLUSION

Literature on mental handicap nursing is limited, literature on community mental handicap nursing is even smaller, and literature on supervision for both is virtually non-existent. A variety of one-to-one and group methods of supervising nurses can be observed within mental handicap teams. These methods not only involve nurses supervising nurses, but also other team members offering supervision support or guidance. Team supervision is often reciprocal and can benefit all professionals working with this particular group of people. It must be pointed out that in all community mental handicap teams, whatever the structure there is a need for nurses to provide some of the supervision of other nurses even though benefits can be gained from a team approach. A system of supervision that may be seen as ideal by one community mental handicap nursing team may not work for another. Equally, a system that works for one nurse may not suit another. Whatever the system of supervision used it must be flexible enough to meet the needs of all nurses and in some teams a variety of approaches are necessary. Sessions should also involve varied styles of supervision so that monotony and boredom do not creep into the activity, but also to ensure that the supervisor explores all aspects of the nurse's practice.

It must be remembered that most community mental handicap nurses were educated and therefore prepared for work in a hospital environment. The change to community work can present many anxieties which need acknowledgement and support of colleagues who have gone through a similar process. Barber and Norman (1987) reiterate the need for 'ongoing professional support so that conflicts may be examined as they arise and relevant on the spot skills can be imparted'. This professional support or supervision must be provided to ensure not only the quantity of a nurse's practice but also its quality.

## REFERENCES

Balcombe, K. (1989) Leading the way, *Nursing Standard*, Issue 16, **3**, 24–6.

Barber, E. and Norman, B. (1987) *Mental Handicap – Facilitating Holistic Care*, Hodder and Stoughton, London.

Bullough, B. *et al.* (1983) *Nursing Issues and Nursing Strategies for the Eighties*, Springer Publishing, New York.

Carr, P. J., Butterworth, C. A. and Hodges, B. E. (1980) *Community Psychiatric Nursing*, Churchill Livingstone, Edinburgh.

Department of Health and Social Security (1974) Report of the Enquiry into South Ockendon Hospital, HMSO, London.

Maclachlan, M. *et al.* (1987) Do the professionals understand?, *Mental Handicap*, **15**(1), 5–7.

Towell, D. (1975) *Understanding Psychiatric Nursing: a sociological analysis of modern psychiatric nursing*, Royal College of Nursing, London.

# CHAPTER TEN

# Issues in the supervision of health visiting practice: an agenda for debate

## Sheila Twinn

The interpretation of the term clinical supervision is generally defined within the context of professional education and training. However some authors argue that this is too restrictive an interpretation and it should be broadened to include the relationship which occurs between practitioners during the process of peer appraisal and review (Butterworth, 1988). This interpretation raises an interesting debate in health visiting which relates not only to the interpretation of professional practice (Robinson, 1987; Twinn, 1989) but also to the significant changes occurring in health visiting intervention (Goodwin, 1988). Indeed it is this type of debate which highlights the significance of the clinical supervision offered to students during their preparation for practice. The following discussion about clinical supervision in health visiting will be considered in that context.

In this particular specialism of community health care clinical supervision occurs in two distinct phases: fieldwork practice and the period of supervised practice. These two components of the health visitor course were introduced following a revision of the curriculum in 1965 and have essentially remained unchanged since that time. Fieldwork practice provides students with an opportunity to rehearse health visiting practice in a protected environment under the guidance of an experienced practitioner who her/himself will have undertaken further education and training for this role. It is perhaps pertinent to note that although the Council for the Education and Training of Health Visitors acknowledged that the initial training offered to Fieldwork Teachers (FWT) had not substantially improved the quality of fieldwork teachers (CETHV, 1975), the revised fieldwork teachers course first introduced in 1975 has also not addressed many of the issues associated with clinical supervision (Fish *et al.*, 1989; Twinn, 1989). The period of supervised practice has been designed as a period of transition which allows the student to consolidate the knowledge and practice skills acquired during fieldwork practice in a working situation. Although different practitioners are responsible for each student during these two discrete periods of the course, it is significant that similar issues emerge pertinent to clinical supervision and one in particular is the interaction between the student and supervisor in the learning environment.

During fieldwork practice it is the FWT (an experienced health visitor who has successfully completed the Community Practice Teacher Course) who has the responsibility of integrating theory and practice and assessing the student's competence to practise. The integration of theory and practice is not only dependent on the supervisor's perception of the relationship between theory and practice but also on the practice available to the student. It is within the context of the relationship of theory and practice that the status of practical knowledge must also be considered and it is only relatively recently that it has been acknowledged that practical knowledge is of equal significance to theoretical knowledge (Schon, 1983). Indeed, these circumstances have led those working in either the theoretical or practical component of professional education to negate the interdependent relationship of each of these components in the education and training of students. It is this phenomenon which has stimulated the creation of a gap between theory and practice, a situation which remains a reality in much of professional education.

The integration of theory and practice will also be influenced by the FWT's interpretation of professional practice. This may be restricted to a narrow range of practice skills or encompass the much broader definition of professional practice which includes the intuition in practice by which practitioners make sense of the unique practice setting (England, 1986; Schon, 1987). It is issues such as these which will influence the student's learning experience as well as the assessment of competence to practise and, in particular, raise three major issues in the supervision of health visitor students: the learning environment, the concept of role modelling and the conflicting demands of teaching and assessing in clinical practice. Although the learning environment must be considered equally in terms of the practice setting and the input provided by the FWT, the quality of the FWT–student interaction plays a major role in influencing the outcome of clinical supervision. However there are specific factors which will influence the quality of this interaction and these include the FWT–student relationship, the standards of practice presented to the student and the opportunity to demonstrate, question and criticize strategies in practice. Perhaps the most significant factor is the ability of the FWT to identify effectively the learning opportunities presented in the student–client–FWT interaction and dialogue. However the opportunity for these processes to occur will be determined in part by the practice setting experienced by the student. Obviously individual professional groups will interpret the term practice setting differently. A useful definition is that provided by Schon (1987) who describes the practice setting in which the student exists as the practicum. The practicum, although resembling the practice world, is free from the pressures, risks and distractions of practice reality and allows the student to learn through actual practice in a protected environment. Nonetheless, three major factors require addressing in relation to this concept in clinical supervision: the extent to which the practicum represents the practice reality, the learning opportunities provided in this setting and the opportunity for the students to rehearse their practice in a sheltered environment.

In order to achieve an effective practicum the setting must obviously represent the essential features of practice and student learning may be inhibited if too many features of the real world or practice are omitted, but learning may be equally inhibited if too many of the practical constraints encountered in actual practice are experienced. Although the guidelines produced by the English National Board (ENB) require the FWT to 'cover a broad range of health visiting practice, provide opportunities for work in a variety of settings and encourage community participation in health education and care' (ENB, 1986, p. 3), in reality much of health visiting practice concentrates on a reactive approach working predominantly with children under five (Goodwin, 1988; DHSS, 1986). It is this type of evidence which questions the extent to which clinical supervision provides the student with the opportunity of exploring the fundamental principles of health visiting practice, in particular the search for health needs (CETHV, 1977).

Although the FWT's understanding of the conceptual origins of health visiting practice will in part determine the learning opportunities provided in the practicum, this will also be influenced by the size and structure of the FWT's caseload. In many health authorities district policy still requires practitioners to carry out routine child health surveillance, which generally restricts the opportunity for group work or facilitating community initiatives in health. The FWT is then dependent upon colleagues for the provision of essential learning opportunities for the student which may once more have implications for the quality of clinical supervision. In addition the FWT's continued professional accountability for a caseload which frequently exceeds that recommended by the Department of Health (Barrell-Davis and Williams, 1984) creates conflict and stress (Dean, 1985), an issue which is discussed in more depth later in the chapter. Finally, the extent to which the practicum provides the student with the opportunity of rehearsing her practice in a partial or protected way while absorbing the appreciative systems and values of health visiting raises another major issue in clinical supervision. Recent studies suggest (Twinn, 1989; Fish *et al.*, 1989) that not only do students spend a considerable amount of time practising without direct supervision but also that the practice briefing and debriefing is essentially descriptive in nature and does not facilitate the process of exploring and analysing different strategies in practice. These findings once more highlight the essential role played by the FWT–student interaction in the learning environment. Another factor which must be considered in the outcome of this interaction is the preparation of the FWT.

Current training for FWTs consists of two parts: a six-week theoretical block and a period of practice under supervision. This supervision is undertaken by a lecturer in health visiting who is also responsible for offering tutorial support and guidance to the student health visitor placed with the FWT completing part two of the course. The level of professional competence demonstrated by the FWT obviously introduces another dimension into the arena of clinical supervision, although it is not intended to explore this dimension in this present discussion. It is anticipated that the training provided for FWTs will enable them effectively to fulfil the role of teacher, counsellor, role model and assessor.

Indeed it is the extent to which the FWT effectively fulfils these roles which raises further issues about clinical supervision. During the six-week course the FWT must develop the expertise to foster the student's learning in the practice setting, particularly by demonstrating, advising, analysing and criticizing strategies of health visiting practice. The extent to which the FWT is competent in this field will in part determine the quality of FWT–student dialogue: a process which is central to the quality of the interaction. However, the processes used to foster learning through practice will also determine the quality of the supervision. Currently, evidence suggests that many FWTs predominantly adopt a model of technical training rather than a model of learning which enables students to develop forms of inquiry by which practitioners adapt their professional knowledge to each unique practice setting.

Another factor which must be taken into consideration when exploring the effectiveness of supervision is the student–FWT relationship. Jarvis and Gibson (1985) argue that a good relationship between the student and FWT is fundamental to the learning environment and directly relates to the needs of the adult learner. Research findings (Dingwall, 1977; Hunkins, 1985) highlight the stress experienced by students while undertaking the health visitor course and the supportive role undertaken by the FWT is essential in helping them to cope with the course. This raises questions as to the extent to which the quality of the supervision is subsequently affected, particularly since a fundamental role of the supervisor is to offer constructive criticism to the student. It is perhaps significant that my research demonstrated that FWTs found this area of practice exceptionally difficult. They stated that they considered an important aspect of their role was to build up the confidence of students rather than adopt a practice characteristic which could be described as destructive. The data provide specific examples of the tendency to make allowance in those students experiencing a difficult time either in their personal life or at college. However, this evidence also raises once more the role of the FWT–student dialogue in clinical supervision.

It is particularly during the dialogue which makes up the briefing prior to and the debriefing following client contact that the processes involved in critically analysing and assessing health visiting strategies adopted during the client–student–FWT interaction are explored. It is this dialogue which provides the FWT with an opportunity to foster learning through practice by reflection-in-action. Fish *et al*. (1989) describe this process as one in which the practitioner:

1.  is alert to the varied characteristics of the placement setting;
2.  is aware of the range of possibilities for action;
3.  draws upon previous relevant experience;
4.  has in mind previously formulated personal theory;
5.  draws upon knowledge of relevant formal theory;
6.  takes account of personal values;
7.  is aware of how these relate to professional frames of reference;
8.  is able to make a professional judgement;
9.  is able to act upon the decision;
10. continually evaluates a decision and its effects.

The findings from this pilot study, as previously described, demonstrate an essentially descriptive dialogue which specifically demonstrates lost teaching and learning opportunities. This not only related to the FWTs who consistently failed to explore the students' level of knowledge but also to the students who accepted what was said to them without asking for further clarification or indeed challenging the statements. In some instances this related specifically to practice issues which raises the question once more of the interpretation and standard of practice presented to students during the period of clinical supervision. It is these issues which highlight not only a fundamental role played by the student–FWT interaction in determining the quality of the supervision but also the need to explore the implications of role modelling during clinical supervision.

The significance of the process of role modelling in clinical supervision has been clearly acknowledged (UKCC, 1986; ENB, 1988; Jarvis and Gibson, 1985). A definition of this concept is provided by Kemper (1968) who describes a role model as 'an individual who possesses certain skills and displays techniques that the individual lacks and from whom, by observation and comparison with his own performance, the individual can learn'. Dotan *et al.* (1986) identified specific factors which influenced whether the clinical supervisor was seen as a role model by general nurses and this included factors such as the extent to which the supervisor regarded teaching the student as important, the extent to which the supervisor's goals matched those of the student and the status of the supervisor amongst her professional colleagues and clients or patients. However, it is significant to note that once again the relationship between the student and the supervisor was highlighted as a significant factor, as indeed were the personality and the interpersonal skills of the supervisor. The attributes of the role model in this study could be categorized into three major groups of traits: professional competence, a humanistic approach and power.

It is interesting that my research in health visiting education reflects similar findings. The data from the student cohort highlighted in particular the significance of the standards of professional practice demonstrated by the FWT and the personality of the FWT. Those FWTs identified as a role model were described as enthusiastic, knowledgeable and interested. There was also a direct correlation between those students who perceived their FWT as role model and those who considered that more time in fieldwork practice would have been beneficial to their learning experience. The data obtained from the FWT cohort, although highlighting an air of resignation and inevitability, also demonstrated the feeling of power associated with the concept of role modelling. In part this was reflected in the intensity of their response to this question in the interview schedule (whether it was negative or positive). However, the power associated with the process was also related to the concern expressed by the FWTs that they should be considered a role model.

The concept was obviously disturbing, with one FWT describing the role as frightening and another stating that she was not prepared to respond to that question. Perhaps one of the most significant findings relates to the difference in perception amongst the FWTs and students as to whether they were or had provided a role model. In only four of the 12 pairs of FWT and students who participated in the in-depth interviews was there an agreement in their perception of whether the FWT was a role model to the student. Indeed it is significant that some FWTs who stated that they considered it an inappropriate role to play were identified by the student sample as a role model. It is this type of evidence which highlights implications for the supervisor of not only their interpretations of practice but also the standard of practice demonstrated in the clinical setting. These issues have particular significance where the supervisor is also responsible for the assessment of competence in practice and the conflict which may arise from the phenomenon provides the focus for the final issue in clinical supervision within the context of health visiting education.

The regulations provided by the ENB (1988) require that the periods of fieldwork and supervised practice are assessed in discrete units of the course. In order to proceed to supervised practice the student must have successfully completed fieldwork practice. Although the ENB provide and require the use of a standardized assessment procedure for supervised practice, this is not the case with fieldwork practice where each individual institution is responsible for producing a framework for assessing the student's competence in practice. Despite the fact that this procedure must be approved during the validation process research has demonstrated the enormous range of criteria used to assess this aspect of professional practice (Twinn, 1989). This highlights the diverse interpretation of professional practice and knowledge which has arisen from a general lack of understanding and application of a conceptual framework for health visiting practice. In turn this has contributed to the conflicting demands experienced by the FWT in his/her role of clinical supervisor.

It has been acknowledged earlier in this chapter that the FWT is required to undertake a variety of roles simultaneously within the practicum. Indeed the practicum demands that the FWT demonstrates a degree of excellence in professional practice which not only includes appropriate knowledge, skills and attitudes but also the intuitive knowing in practice by which practitioners make sense of the practice setting to inform professional judgements and determine strategies in practice. In addition, the FWT must provide a learning resource for the student and take responsibility for assessing the student's competence in practice. It has been argued that role conflict occurs when existing role expectations are contradictory or mutually exclusive and it is apparent that the role expectations of a facilitator, role model and assessor are not necessarily compatible and may indeed be contradictory. In addition the FWT remains professionally accountable to his/her clients, colleagues and health authority.

The role of assessor is one of particular significance in the clinical supervision of health visitor students. Although FWTs acknowledge their specific responsibility in the area of student education and training (Twinn, 1989), previous research has identified not only their concern about their ability to undertake this role but also the finding that this is the least popular aspect of fieldwork teaching (Chapman, 1978; Dean, 1985). This may be attributed in part to the responsibility associated with this role which particularly relates to the issue of failing a student. However, it also raises once more the issue of offering constructive criticism to the student, another aspect of fieldwork practice in which practitioners experience difficulty despite the process being fundamental to clinical supervising. Another issue which must be considered within this context is the extent to which the assessment of the student reflects the teaching and learning experience provided for the student. Although some FWTs acknowledge that the student's performance directly or indirectly reflects their input during the practicum the concept of role modelling implicitly raises issues which require addressing by those involved generally in clinical supervision. A question which relates specifically to health visiting education is whose practice is the FWT assessing, her own or the students?

This question directly raises another issue reflecting the conflicting demands made upon the FWT: the standard of professional practice presented to the student. The implications of the FWT's standard of practice in relation to role modelling have been previously discussed, however fieldwork teaching also demands that the FWT is an expert in teaching. This requires the FWT to straddle two professions and be expert in both (Jarvis and Gibson, 1985). Although this is not unique to health visiting, it highlights the demands that are made upon practitioners in keeping up to date with the contemporary issues and developments in two discrete professional groups. It is perhaps significant that research findings suggest that managers and practitioners currently place a greater emphasis on in-service training in the practice of health visiting than teaching (Maggs and Purr, 1990).

The requirement for the FWT to act as a learning resource for students raises further concerns for clinical supervision, in particular this relates to the amount of time the FWT devotes to fieldwork teaching. The significance that students attach to the amount of time that the FWT is able or prepared to give to the teaching role has been clearly identified. This issue in itself creates conflict for FWTs as often they are aware that they have insufficient time to allocate to the student if the standard of practice offered to clients is not to be compromised.

One other area of possible conflict which requires addressing in relation to the learning resource offered by the FWT to the student is associated with the concept of the learning bind. Schon (1987) describes a learning bind as an episode when the student and the teacher fail to notice that they have missed each other's meaning in the interpretation of a practice situation. Indeed Schon argues that the ability to escape from the learning bind depends equally on the teacher's ability to reflect on the teacher–student dialogue as well as recognizing that it is not necessarily the student's failure to grasp a teaching point. In health visiting supervision this issue has specific relevance in the interpretation of professional practice. The conflicting paradigms of practice have led students specifically to describe their frustration when their perception of client need has differed from that of the FWT. It is this type of debate which may create conflict for the supervisor and have particular implications for the assessment process.

One other factor which must be considered in clinical supervision is the experience students bring with them to the learning environment. In health visiting students enter the practicum with a wide range of personal and professional experience and very different perceptions of health visiting practice. The extent to which the student benefits from the learning experience will in part depend on the student's willingness 'to step into' the practicum, but by participating in this process students frequently experience feelings of loss which may include loss of control, competence and confidence. This in turn leads to feelings of vulnerability which may be demonstrated in the student by overt defensiveness. These feelings of loss may be particularly exacerbated in a process which requires a practitioner to assume student status despite paradoxically being required to adopt a practitioner role in a learning experience. It is this type of evidence which highlights the need for the FWT to demonstrate a sensitivity and an understanding of the requirements of the adult learner. Although the FWT–student relationship emerges as a fundamental element influencing the quality and outcome of clinical supervision there are specific factors associated with the three major issues identified at the beginning of the chapter which directly relate to the education and training needs of FWTs.

The effectiveness of the learning environment is dependent not only on the skills of the FWT but also the interpretation of professional practice presented to the student. In order to develop expertise within this context it is essential that FWTs consider their own theoretical basis for professional practice. In health visiting this involves FWTs re-examining the conceptual origins of practice and developing a conceptual framework for practice which will enable them to analyse the relationship between theory and practice and the different kinds of models of practice which develop in the practice setting. It is this type of process which is essential if the student is going to use the practicum effectively to rehearse his/her practice. However, the FWT will need the opportunity to develop and practise these skills; a factor which is not considered in the current Community Practice Teachers Course.

The influence of the role model in determining the outcome of clinical supervision must also be considered in relation to the education and training of FWTs. The FWT will need to explore his/her own particular abilities, capacities, skills, assumptions and values and how these concepts influence the interpretation of professional practice. The FWT will need to consider whether his/her practice incorporates the more abstract components of competent professional practice, in particular whether the role model incorporates the intuitive knowing in practice which is fundamental in determining effective strategies in practice. Once again the FWT will need the opportunity to develop these skills, particularly in self-awareness and reflection. It is also essential that the process of reflection not only occurs after practice but also while in the midst of practice if the practitioner is to develop the expertise to enable the student to learn through practice. These processes are not experienced in the current courses.

The conflicting demands of teaching and assessing in clinical practice also raises questions about the needs of the FWT. These include issues such as exploring the difference between practising and supervising another person's practice, how the complexities of practice might be used to enable the student to learn more effectively through practice and, most significantly, how the complex nature of the assessment of practice relates to the supervision of the student. It is questions such as these which illustrate the inadequacy of the current courses in preparing practitioners for their vital role in student supervision and highlight the commonality of these issues in the clinical supervision of students from many different professional groups.

## REFERENCES

Barrell-Davis, L. and Williams, W. M. (1984) *Health Visitor*, Manpower Survey, 1979–1981, *Health Visitor*, 1984, **57**(1), 9–14.

Butterworth, T. (1988) Breaking the boundaries, *Nursing Times*, 23 Nov., **84**(47), 36–39.

CETHV (1975) Fifth Report, 1969–1974, CETHV.

CETHV (1977) An Investigation into the Principles of Health Visiting, CETHV.

Chapman, V. (1978) An exploratory case study of the role of the FWT, M.Sc. thesis, University of Surrey, unpublished.

Dean, A. (1985) *Prelude to Practice*, RCN, London.

Department of Health and Social Security (1986) *Neighbourhood Nursing – a focus for care*, HMSO, London.

Dingwall, R. (1977) *The Social Organisation of Health Visitor Training*, Croom Helm, London.

Dotan, M. *et al.* (1986) Role models in nursing, *Nursing Times Occ. Papers*, 12 Feb., **82**(3), 55–57.

England, H. (1986) *Social Work as Art: making sense for good practice*, Allen & Unwin, London.

English National Board for Nursing Midwifery and Health Visiting (1988) Health Visitor and Related Courses Rules, Regulations and Notes on Guidance syllabuses, ENB.

142        *Supervision of health visiting practice*

English National Board (1986) Guidelines for Fieldwork Teacher Placements, ENB.

Fish, D., Twinn, S. and Purr, B. (1989) *How to Enable Learning through Professional Practice*, West London Press, London.

Goodwin, S. (1988) *Whither Health Visiting?* Health Visitors Association, London.

Hunkins, I. (1985) Counselling needs of students, *Health Visitor*, **58**, Mar., 69–70.

Jarvis, P. and Gibson, S. (1985) *The Teacher Practitioner in Nursing, Midwifery and Health Visiting*, Croom Helm, London.

Kemper, T. D. (1968) Reference groups, socialisation and achievement, *American Sociological Review*, **33**, 35–45.

Maggs, C. and Purr, B. (1990) *An Exploration of the Continual Preparation of Fieldwork and Practical Work Teachers in England*, Ashdale Press, London.

Robinson, J. (1987) *Health Visiting Theory – Where do we go from here in Thinking About Health Visiting?*, Thomas Coram Research Unit, University of London Institute of Education.

Schon, D. A. (1983) *The Reflective Practitioner*, Basic Books, New York.

Schon, D. A. (1987) *Educating the Reflective Practitioner*, Jossey-Bass Publishers, San Francisco.

Twinn, S. F. (1989) *Change and Conflict in Health Visiting Practice: Dilemmas in the assessment of competence of student Health Visitors*, Ph.D. thesis, London University Institute of Education, unpublished.

UKCC (1986) *Project 2000*, UKCC, London.

# CHAPTER ELEVEN

# Child protection: health visiting and supervision

## *Robert Nettleton*

. . . we believe that, however experienced the practitioners might be, child abuse work is sufficiently complex and demanding as to require, invariably, good supervision. (*A Child in Mind*, London Borough of Greenwich, 1987)

The development of supervision in nursing can be seen to be generated from a number of diverse influences both within and outside the profession—as related by other contributors to this volume. However, the protection of children from parental mistreatment is a concern that has a particular impact. It is a concern voiced in the media, the professions and government, stimulated by notable incidents of what Dingwall, Eekelaar and Murray (1983) term 'agency failures': that is, by the deaths of abused children which have been subject to special inquiry reports or apparently 'over-zealous' intervention as in the case of Cleveland (DHSS, 1988a).

Child abuse inquiries have stimulated considerable political and professional response. In particular the Beckford report (London Borough of Brent, 1985) and the Carlile report (London Borough of Greenwich, 1987) link failures in the performance of the health visitors and social workers concerned, with inadequacies in the professional supervision provided by the field workers' superiors. In its critical account of the role of the health visitor, the Beckford report states, 'The aspect that has most troubled us has been the question of supervision'. The Senior Nurse told the panel of inquiry that the health visitors under her supervision 'were expected to recognise their own areas of weakness and of doubt about their responses to individual cases, and to approach her for guidance and assistance'. In contradistinction to this approach the report states of supervision, 'It must be proactive, and not just reactive' (p. 143). In 1987 the Minister of State for Health asked the Standing

Nursing and Midwifery Advisory Committee (SNMAC) in the Department of Health and Social Security (DHSS) to form a working party,

> To produce guidance for senior nurses who in the course of their professional duties supervise, monitor and assist in training of nurses, health visitors and midwives in matters relating to child abuse, including child sexual abuse. (Press Release)

The report produced with the title 'Child Protection: Guidance for Senior Nurses, Health Visitors and Midwives' (DHSS, 1988b) takes into account the need for 'providing professional advice and for the supervision of staff' (p. 6) in a variety of specialisms and contexts. In terms of developing a model of supervision this is of particular importance. The Beckford report (London Borough of Greenwich, 1987) shows scant regard for the particular context of health visiting. The latter places a strong emphasis upon the importance of supervision in child abuse work (chapter 30). However, while its detailed discussion relates to the role of the social worker in the Carlile case, it states that supervision applies 'with like effect' to health visitors and their managers.

This can be seen to be a misleading over-simplification of the case in what the Chairman of the SNMAC working party acknowledges to be a sensitive and complex area.

It is probably impossible to define 'supervision' too rigidly for all disciplines and settings, as each can be expected to have its own understandings and uses of such terms. 'Speaking a suitable language' requires that a language be learned, understood and used in a community of shared meaning and is a necessary component of a 'safe professional apparatus' (Butterworth, 1988) which is being demanded for dealing with child abuse. Munsen (1976) notes that supervision in social work is as old as the profession itself, but the term is used in a wide variety of ways. Parsloe and Hill (DHSS, 1978) have noted that social workers use the word supervision 'in a peculiar way'. On the grounds that it may be a fair assumption that each group in nursing uses the word 'supervision' in a relatively peculiar way, it may be helpful to focus on how supervision is understood in one grouping—that of health visiting.

'Supervision' is not part of the language of health visiting, but this is not to say that supervision does not take place, is not recognized as a need, or valued in practice. The remainder of this chapter focuses upon field work observation made by the author during a current research project which thus provides accounts of the practice of health visiting which may contribute to the development of a model for supervision.

Part of the context of supervision in this domain are the varying 'ideologies of child abuse' (Parton, 1985) and the position of health visiting in this context (Dingwall *et al.*, 1983). Parton (1985) summarizes these ideologies as medical, traditional social welfare and radical social welfare ideologies. He follows Newberger and Bourne (1977) in suggesting two central issues in constructing policies and practices towards families in crisis: family autonomy versus coercive intervention and compassion versus control. Social policy and professional response can be understood as attempts to resolve the dilemmas represented by these polarities conditioned by the ideologies of child abuse which carry most influence. These themes emerge in the supervision of health visitors in the nature of the health visitor inter-client relationship, professional autonomy, accountability and the role of management. Thus differing prospectives concerning the nature of child abuse have a bearing upon understanding the nature of supervision. Put crudely, the performance of a health visitor may be viewed in terms of her individual adequacy (or pathology), the environment or system in which she operates, or as being in need of liberation from an oppressive hierarchical social structure.

## FORMS OF SUPPORT AND SUPERVISION

Health visitors offer an unsolicited service to a largely well population which includes all families where there are children under the age of five. The SNMAC report recognizes that work with abused or neglected children will generally be only a part of the duties of community-based nurses (DHSS, 1988a, p. 13). However, a number of studies indicate that dealing with child abuse is anxiety provoking or stressful for health visitors (Gough and Hingley, 1988; Appleby, 1987; Bennett and Dauncey, 1986). The main sources of support for dealing with child abuse take the form of informal peer group support (e.g. in the health visitors' office) and managerial support. Appleby (1987) adds to these sources support groups of which there are a number of accounts in the literature (Spicer, 1980; Vizard, 1983; Milne, Walker and Bamford, 1987; Goldblatt, 1988; Dare and Lansberry, 1988; Richardson and Dunn, 1987).

## PEER GROUP SUPPORT

Current field work research by the author confirms that peer group support is highly valued by health visitors. One health visitor, who felt good peer group support was vital, related what she believed were the qualities of 'good' support. 'A trusting non-competitive group. You need to feel confident that if you disclose a weakness it is accepted by the group as normal. If you make mistakes, you are personally supported by the group—even if you're in the wrong. That is what you need. You haven't got to feel threatened by any one member.' This health visitor's experience of peer group support was very positive. Her office developed a 'mutual appreciation society' which enabled them to cope better with very distressing situations. However the office environment may not always be so supportive.

> I think it depends on how your colleagues are feeling. If they're feeling down you tend to feel a bit down as well with them, but if everyone's happy it's great, you know. You are affected whoever is around when you're working.

Another health visitor related a situation in which 'everyone was talking in the office but no-one could afford to listen, they had so much of their own anxiety to deal with'. She went on to observe that, like family, work colleagues are not so much chosen as thrust upon us. Supportive relationships do not just happen.

This can be appreciated from the history of primary health care teams. McIntosh and Dingwall (1978) have pointed out the assumption made by middle managers in the 1970s that practice attachment and team work were synonymous, thus viewing difficulties as personal problems of individuals rather than structural processes. Smith and Ames (1976) have also observed that formation of a team does not necessarily equate with sharing responsibility for decisions in such a way as to be perceived as supportive.

Health visitors carry individual 'caseloads' although certain tasks are commonly shared. The extent to which professional identity is seen in individualistic, highly autonomous terms influences the capacity of shared decision making. However, it has been noted that dealing with child abuse can induce a sense of isolation which can endanger good practice.

One group of health visitors endorsed the value to them of peer group support, but complained that 'there's no place on the stats form for it'. Later a health visitor pointed out that there was indeed a category for 'face-to-face liaison with colleagues'. It seems that not only do health visitors need to be given permission to engage in supportive activities, but they also need to be able to take permission for themselves.

It would seem that both personal and situational factors need to be taken into account. Talking with colleagues may raise anxiety as much as reduce it, for example, if the situation is seen as more dangerous, or solutions are proposed which are different to the one the health visitor would feel happy to pursue.

> You haven't got to feel threatened by any one member. It only takes

one to be judgemental and uncommunicative . . . It comes down to personal qualities, plus applying your health visiting skills to the group you work with. By that I mean identifying a concern weighing them down and giving them the opportunity to use you.

In a research interview this health visitor, when asked, 'If you have one isolated or uncommunicative member does it affect the group?', replied, 'Yes, but it doesn't stop the support—you get breakaway groups'. This illustrates the tendency towards what Smith and Ames (1976) term clique formation which, while possibly functional for the group, makes the emergence of at least one 'professional isolate' probable. Thus, informal peer group support, while highly valued, has its limitations. The most supportive environment may not extend to all group members. The reduction of anxiety is not always desirable:

> We would positively say, 'Well, I think you did a really good job.'
> Mind . . . we used to say you could probably rationalize anything . . .

Dealing with child abuse can produce its own dynamics of isolation and paralysis. This is illustrated by an experienced health visitor who valued highly the support of her colleagues and her manager. Amongst the professional network—the social worker, the school, the community drug team, probation and the GP—this health visitor was isolated. 'I'll leave it to you', said the GP. He had indirectly communicated to her 'in code' certain diagnostic information concerning one family member which she felt added to the risk to the children. However, she did not feel able to share this with anyone. The other agencies disputed what action should or could be taken and 'meanwhile you are keeping an eye . . .'

> Jane [the mother] comes to see me—because I'm older than the social worker—she seems to accept me better . . . I get forced into it by the mother—I'm trying to withdraw because I don't think its my role . . .

> I don't know what she'll do if he [the cohabitee] goes into prison . . . you never know when she's telling the truth . . .

The voluntary basis of the health visitor–client relationship characterized by a sense of continuing (rather than episodic) responsibility, with relatively little professional power, places the health visitor close to her client. While her anxieties are focused on risks to the children, who is the de facto client? The health visitor's isolation and vulnerability seem to mirror that of Jane. But who is the most 'powerful' and what is the power for? In this case the health visitor is depleted and cut off from her usual supplies, seemingly unable to stem the flow, with no confidence that it reaches the children, the objects of her concern.

## MANAGERIAL SUPPORT

At the beginning of this chapter it was noted that the Beckford inquiry report advocated that health visitor managers should be proactive rather than reactive in the provision of supervision. On the other hand Dingwall *et al.* (1983) believe that the very existence of health visiting rests upon the voluntaristic nature of the health visitor–client relationship, an arm's length relationship with the state and weak management. They nonetheless believe that lack of public accountability is a problem which requires the strengthening of the supervisory powers of 'first-line managers'. However, as a Director of Nursing Services pointed out forcibly to the present writer health visitors are considered 'first line managers in their own right'. The ambiguity of health visitors towards the support and supervision has been discussed. What are the qualities of managers which are valued by health visitors, and which enable managers to carry out their role?

Dingwall *et al.* (1983) believe that the principal determinants of service quality in health visiting are the individual conscience and skills of the field worker who makes the judgements which nursing officers are obliged to trust.

One reason for this is that the work of the health visitor is 'invisible' and quality cannot be controlled by inspection of a tangible product or direct observational surveillance. A manager in post for about one year related this to the author:

> It's not enough just to know how the injury occurred or what action was taken—I need the whole situation. There is a distance between being involved as a health visitor and being a manager. The health visitor has got the whole picture in here [her head] of her contact with the family. To supervise health visiting I've got to have as much knowledge as I possibly can—otherwise its just, 'Oh, fill in the review form, put them in the system, visit once a month'. You could put that on a piece of paper—its not really management.

Here is an indication of the skills required for supervision to do with enabling the health visitor to communicate her knowledge, and to assimilate it meaningfully. There is also the recognition of levels of supervisory activity. The manager acknowledges a dichotomy between a task-centred, rule-following approach and a more person-centred approach.

This vignette also indicates that there are various methods of communication which may be employed in the supervisory relationship. The 'system' refers to a monitoring system whereby children considered to be 'at risk' or of particular concern are reviewed regularly. The SNMAC Child Protection guidelines (DHSS, 1988b) indicate the value of a coordinating monitoring system. In the author's health authority children who have been abused, are considered at risk or are of particular concern to health visitors can be placed in the system, activating the distribution of monitor forms at intervals determined by the field health visitor and her senior nurse. A senior nurse interviewed by the author described the purpose of the system.

> It is a method for ensuring that the families who have difficulties and children whom the health visitors (HVs) are concerned about, are monitored on a regular basis by the HV and the manager. It is not that the children themselves benefit directly, but it's for the benefit of the HV to discuss ideas of ways forward and draw on someone with greater experience than them. It's a way of HVs bringing forward cases—a forum for the HV to discuss different problems without feeling they are failing by raising the issues. I think it is quite important—we are professionals in our own right and have to be seen to be managing our own caseloads and yet it can be difficult especially if you are not experienced, you can feel lost if you are not supported.

The pattern of monitoring systems across the country is difficult to determine not least due to changes in management structures. Such systems, although of value, have their limitations. Confusion can arise from terminology, such as 'at risk register'. It is easy to confuse a monitoring or supervisory tool for the Child Protection Register administered by the Social Services Department of the local authority (or in some cases the NSPCC), under the auspices of an inter-agency Joint Child Protection Committee.

Secondly, too much should not be asked of such systems. They cannot themselves ensure the safety of children. The Beckford inquiry report (London Borough of Brent, 1985) notes that the Health Authority in which Jasmine Beckford died had such a 'Health Visitors Concern' list.

Thirdly, such systems can be open to criticisms concerning the values they may embody. Who is being 'monitored' or 'supervised' by whom? Is it the child and parents or the health visitor? Recognition of this question is implicit in the senior nurse's account above.

This issue relates to a fourth limitation connected to the 'disease model' of prevention of child abuse. In this chapter the focus is upon the process rather than the content of supervision. Suffice it to say, the 'risk factor' approach needs to be recognized explicitly as an exercise in value judgements. From the health visitor's perspective such systems are valued as a means to an end. The danger of a system becoming an end in itself is exemplified by the comment of a health visitor who said in the context of support and supervision that one might say things to a colleague which would not be said to a senior nurse because 'she would just say "write a report" '. Thus rather than assisting the health visitor, systems may prove irksome. This is consistent with the observation by Smith and Ames (1976) of the conflict experienced by professionals working in bureaucratic organizations who may find them not conducive to professional support. They suggest that emphasis on bureaucratic procedures may correspond to a lack of professional resources for consultation. Thus while the organization may be highly efficient at dealing with problems subject to administrative solutions, it may seem 'barren of expertise and moral sensitivity' when difficult, fateful decisions have to be made. It has been noted that a health visitor is powerfully placed to undermine an approach which does not win her support and appreciation, due to the 'invisible' nature of her work. More positively, when asked how she coped with a worrying situation the health visitor said:

> I talked to my senior nurse. I can phone her and off-load—not just write a report . . . by telling someone else it makes you feel better . . . and everyone is supportive in the office.

One senior nurse interviewed by the author expressed the balance of responsibility in supervision.

> The spectre of a child dying from neglect or abuse must be every nursing officer's nightmare. One of the things I hope I have made reasonably clear is that I have the responsibility to give the support and know about the cases and help them [HVs] make decisions, but that they also have a responsibility to let me know because they have the responsibility of managing the caseloads. I have a responsibility to enquire and to be aware and we need to discuss and come to a mutual decision about how to proceed. I also need to be aware of the policy and procedures and ensure that they are adhered to.

From this it can be seen that supervisory relationships do not so much depend upon a simple concentration of power up the hierarchy but are characterized by mutual dependence and trust. The health visitors' access to a home rests on this voluntaristic basis and is thus highly (though not exclusively) relationship focused (Robinson, 1982); likewise managers are obliged to trust their field staff for their accounts of their activities. On the other hand health visitors characteristically initiate and sustain relationships on the principle of the search for health needs and managers themselves can be proactive in providing supervision and support. This does not occur in a social and moral vacuum. All are subject to norms which indicate often unclearly the rights and duties of parents and professionals with respect to the needs of children. Policies, procedures, guidelines, systems, professional and organizational structures provide the visible normative context. They would seem to fulfil their normative function to the extent that they allow trust to be maintained on realistic foundations.

Dealing with conflict of opinion in decision making illuminates the nature of managerial supervision in health visiting. When asked, 'Did you ever have a conflict with a manager as an experienced HV?' a health visitor compared her experience of two senior nurses:

> Well Hilary just reacted—She was action-wise without really reflecting on it. But when I had Gill that was different—she was so superb—she would get you to the right point—she would help you to make a decision. You would come to a decision but if you were really stuck she would say, I think this. She was non-directive and you learned in the process, and sometimes there wasn't a decision and that was okay. Hilary is very clear thinking—she goes straight to the nub very quickly, but she doesn't always take you with her. It can feel to you like it's an arbitrary decision and you don't always learn from it—although it may well be a very good decision in itself.

From the perspective of senior nurses in the author's research direct conflict with field staff seemed minimal. This seemed to be achieved by heavy reliance on compromise.

> I can remember once when a health visitor wasn't happy with what I was saying . . . I thought we would probably get the same outcome anyway. I think we agreed she [the HV] wouldn't go to the GP [about it], but give it another three days . . . I think the health visitor is a professional and can make the decision as well as I.

Does such a reliance upon compromise leave the door open to collusion? Responsibility for decision making seems to be acknowledged to rest both with the individual field health visitor *and* with the senior nurse. This apparent contradiction seems to resolve itself in compromise. Thus when asked,

> Where does the responsibility lie for taking initiative between the health visitor and the senior nurse?

a senior nurse said,

> In practice it is with the Senior Nurse, but you have got to make the climate right—you have got to make yourself accessible and acceptable to them—it's a dual responsibility.

And later, when asked,

> Where does responsibility lie for decision making?

She answered,

> I think it's with me. When I was a health visitor I thought it was with me then.

Thus when this manager did over-rule and direct a member of staff she described it as exceptional:

> It doesn't fit in with how I would usually deal with it. But I needed to take action on behalf of the child.

The situation was also unusual because to the senior nurse at least the line of action required was clear cut whereas far more commonly situations lie in grey areas.

> What made the conflict alright was the relief that a long study problem was coming to a head and her [the health visitor's] internal conflicts were over-ruled by me. She said to me, 'What a relief'.

Given the importance of informal peer group support, one might expect a manager to take this into account when difficulties arise. A senior nurse described her role.

> I have long-term goals—to work quietly to resolve those sort of problems. I do not believe in confrontation unless absolutely necessary; it sometimes causes more problems. I feel I do have skills in manoeuvring people in ways that will sort things out—not dramatic but will cause the right result—it's over a longer period of time. There is one clinic with a lot of clashes, bickering about workloads, etc. I put in an HV who would be able to cope and I addressed the workload problems directly and they are working much better together despite continuing workload stresses.

She also described an initiative to facilitate support and supervision at another clinic.

> At first at one of the clinics I couldn't even get the HVs to leave their desks until after a few weeks. The discussion was at the end of staff meetings and people drifted off to do other things while it was going on. It was less like that at other clinics. It was always at the end. I wanted all the HVs to listen to all the cases. So, then I *began* with cases. I don't always do this now but I have established the priority

and it is working now. If it ever slips I'll bring it back to the top of the agenda. It's part of team building—the staff in a clinic pulling together in the same direction—not just individuals. I think it is very important because some work in quite isolated situations.

The context in which management supervision may be said to take place may typically include clinic meetings, locality staff meetings, occasional one-to-one consultations on a planned basis or telephone discussions, particularly in a crisis. Preparation for and attendance at child protection case-conferences and court proceedings also involve the senior nurse. In addition to these formats and the use of monitoring systems, there would seem to be scope for developing methods of communicating case-related material. In the author's own practice genograms have proved useful in depicting complex family compositions and systemic questions, such as those in Neuman's (1982) systems model of nursing, in elucidating the patterns of resistance to change in chronic situations of concern. However, development of methods of supervision needs to take into account existing processes in order to be incorporated into a coherent model.

## INTER-AGENCY ASPECTS OF SUPERVISION

A significant aspect of the managerial role in support and supervision of health visitors dealing with child abuse is in its inter-agency aspects. Peer group support can and does extend beyond the health visitor's office to supportive relationships with social workers and GPs.

> Sometimes talking with the social workers was very helpful to me—and having to understand the social worker's role so that you knew what sort of things you could off-load to them.

The implementation of 'core groups' as advocated by the DHSS (1988c) document 'Working Together' formalizes the joint working of front-line workers in child protection cases. The author's experience suggests there is much to be gained from sharing consultancy skills across agencies and professions.

However, the differing places occupied by social service departments and health visitors in the child protection system predispose to certain tensions. When the former work under the principle of 'minimal necessary intervention' and the latter under the principle of 'the search for health needs', the stage is set for tensions to surface as in the following example.

The mother was aged 16 with an occasional co-habitee. She lived at several addresses, sometimes with friends and sometimes with her boyfriend and was occasionally homeless. The health visitor was very concerned that a young baby was not being adequately cared for at the level of feeding, clothing, protection from cold and general safety, especially with regard to the mother's violent co-habitee. The health visitor made considerable efforts to trace the mother and baby. Also her clinic attendance was minimal and she did not keep appointments to which she had agreed. The health visitor had placed the child's name on Child Observation System immediately and had also referred to Social Services.

> One of the worst things was the Social Services—I felt no-one would believe me. I thought something was bound to happen sooner or later. I referred to social services but they kept saying, 'What's the social work task?' I thought it was obvious—the baby was at risk and my concern was prevention. It was like I had to prove something to them. Eventually the case was accepted and allocated when the baby was two months old. Then everything changed. I think partly it was that they got a new social worker—I know they had been understaffed. But she [the social worker] was really good. Before this they just sent a letter to her [the mother] and said they got no reply. Well, they wouldn't since she was moving about. I was out there asking in her friend's flat and asking the caretaker, 'Have you seen this girl who looks like . . . with a small baby?' At first he would say no but then when I said I was the HV and that I just wanted to let her know about the clinic so the baby could be weighed he said, 'Oh yes, try that one'.

The case is taken up by the Senior Nurse:

> The mother disappeared for three weeks and when I got in touch with Social Services the senior social worker said 'what more do you want me to do?' I said we should go to the police, but she disagreed. I felt it wouldn't have been harmful to the relationship [with the mother]. Because I didn't leave, she agreed that if the mother hadn't turned up after another 3 days I should 'phone the police. The HV had kept in touch with me. We had agreed she would try to find the mother and baby and she made every possible effort. I was concerned, one, for the safety of the child and, two, for the anxiety of the HV. So I decided I should take some responsibility. The social worker was quite happy to let us shoulder the responsibility without accepting the responsibility herself because there was no evidence of actual harm to the child. We sometimes say 'well what do you want—an injury?' That's the difference between us—we are preventative, whereas the Social Services respond to a crisis, to an actual injury or to evidence of neglect. There is a difference between Social Services and us about where we feel they should come in and when they will do so. For

example we make 'information only' referrals for future use or to indicate that we have done what we could.

This example indicates the supportive role of the senior nurse and some of the stresses particular to the position of the health visitor in the inter-agency system for protecting children at risk. Dingwall *et al.* (1983) describe this system as being underpinned by the liberal compromise, analogous to a separation of power in the state. Supervision in child protection needs to uphold the legitimate concerns of health visitors in the multi-agency arena, especially taking into account the deliberate avoidance of coercion in favour of principles of 'stimulating awareness', 'facilitating' and 'influencing' (CETHV, 1977), with respect to the health needs of children and policies which affect them. These principles simultaneously place health visitors closer to clients, allowing them to search for health needs, and make them vulnerable to shifting of responsibility by more distant child protection agencies. It is all too easy for the health visitor to mirror the apparent powerlessness of dangerous families to change, and their incipient violence to become reflected in inter-agency conflict. It is a key function of supervision to be aware of these processes, to identify their effects and to enable field staff to carry out their own role effectively in the inter-agency context.

## DEVELOPING A MODEL IN A CHANGING ENVIRONMENT

At a time when change can seem to be a rare constant in professional life, a model of supervision must take into account such policies. The Health Visitors' Association (1987) document 'A Stitch in Time . . .' focuses on the changes in management structure linked to the implementation of general management (Griffiths Report, DHSS, 1984) and the Community Nursing Review (Cumberlege Report, DHSS, 1986). The HVA document states that two pre-requisites for any management structure for providing a safe, effective and efficient service are clearly defined channels of communication, and lines of accountability with mechanisms which include all staff. These pre-requisites are brought into particularly sharp focus in the area of supervision and support of health visitors dealing with child abuse. Notwithstanding the ambivalence with which the role of nursing officer has been regarded, the management structures emanating from the Salmon (Ministry of Health, 1966) and Mayston (DHSS, 1969) Reports provided a clear line of professional and managerial accountability. However, the implementation of the Griffiths Report recommendations (DHSS, 1984) has to a greater or lesser extent split these functions. In addition, neighbourhood nursing teams of district nurses, health visitors and school nurses brought into being in response to the Cumberlege Report (DHSS, 1986) are not necessarily managed by a health visitor. In these circumstances both the HVA (1987) and the Nurse Advisors to the Community Nursing Review Team (Carpentier-Alting and Brown, 1986) assert that provisions must be made for professional health visiting advice and support for health visitors dealing with child abuse cases. There remains scope for variability, not to say confusion concerning professional accountability and the meaning of 'supervision'.

The appointment of Senior Nurse Advisors (Child Abuse) as advocated by the SNMAC report Child Protection (DHSS, 1988b) may be part of the response to this need. It may be that a more collegiate rather than hierarchical approach may facilitate development of a pattern of supervision which is understood in terms of advice and consultation rather than management. Where this occurs issues of accountability need to be clarified and defined accordingly. The Carlile inquiry report (London Borough of Greenwich, 1987) states emphatically that 'Consultation may conveniently be used to supplement, but never to replace [professional and managerial] supervision'. The members of the Commission believed it to be 'perfectly practicable for one person to perform the task of good manager and good supervisor to the same members of staff'. Whether or not this is so in a changing ethos of managerialism flowing from the Griffiths Report (DHSS, 1984) and the National Health Service and Community Care Act, 1990, supportive supervisory relationships need to be maintained.

Goodwin (1988) has confronted the need for health visiting to respond positively to multi-dimensional change. She re-emphasizes the voluntaristic nature of the health visitor–client relationship stating that an imperative for change is the recognition of

> the need for more participative and less directive relationships with clients, and developing group and community approaches.

She acknowledges that there is a continuing role for health visitors in child health promotion while noting that practice has become trapped by traditional home visiting and a child health centred model. Goodwin suggests that a future framework for practice should retain a universal unrestricted provision which avoids stigmatization. At the same time, targeting client groups is required to meet today's health needs within the present constraints on services. She asks, 'What about child abuse . . .?', and acknowledges 'that we can't be sure of that now'.

A child protection perspective might suggest that health visiting should not be conceived simply as a service to 'families with children under five'. While Goodwin suggests that parental needs should be assessed and responded to as legitimate in their own right, the reality of child abuse reminds us that we also need to assess and respond to the needs of children as legitimate in their own right and not only in relation to their parents. Supervision in child protection work always needs to keep in view the primary need of the most vulnerable individuals within families, groups and committees, recognizing that children too are clients.

## CONCLUSION

In the foregoing account of health visiting, child abuse has been identified as a most demanding aspect of professional practice. Child protection is defined in a normative framework, which is by no means fully consistent or static. A model of supervision needs to take into account the particularities of the professional context, for example, the voluntary nature of health visitor–client relationship. In other settings common features of child protection work, such as inter-professional cooperation, have particular manifestations. For example, for the school nurse the relationship with teaching staff and their particular orientations are critical. In paediatric wards dealing with parents gives rise to tensions when they may not be allowed to participate in the care of their children under the same conditions fostered by the ward's philosophy of care for children and families in general.

Professional accountability is brought into sharp relief by the glare of public attention upon the child protection worker. It highlights that aspirations to autonomy cannot safely be equated with isolation. A safe professional model for practice does not consist only of policies, procedures and management structures and systems, but these should underpin supportive supervisory relationships. Protection implies vulnerability. The anxiety of health visitors and others dealing with child abuse indicates the everyday reality of vulnerability. Perhaps what is needed is 'Protection with autonomy' (DHSS, 1978). In this concept, autonomy is related to an implied interdependency. A model of child protection supervision needs to be sensitive enough to hear the voices of the most vulnerable, and to magnify them so that children and those who have their welfare closest to their hearts can be heard and protected.

## REFERENCES

Appleby, F. M. (1987) Professional support and the role of support groups. *Health Visitor Manual*, **60**, 77–78.
Bennett, V. and Dauncey, J. (1986) Significant events for health visitors during practice, *Health Visitor*, April, **59**, 103–104.
Butterworth, C. A. (1988) Breaking the boundaries: New endeavours in community nursing. (Inaugural lecture) May 1988, University of Manchester, Department of Nursing.

Carpentier-Alting, S. and Brown, P. (1986) Letter to the 'Health Visitor' by Nurse Advisors to the Community Nursing Review Team, *Health Visitor*, **59**, 327.

CETHV (1977) An investigation into the principles of health visiting, Council for the Education and Training of Health Visiting, London.

Dare, J. and Lansberry, C. (1988) Health visitor support groups, *Health Visitor*, Feb., **61**, 41–42.

DHSS (1969) Report of DHSS Working Party on Management Structure in the Local Authority Nursing Services (Mayston Report), DHSS.

DHSS (1978) Social Service Teams: The Practitioner's view. (P. Parsloe and M. Hill), HMSO, London.

DHSS (1984) Health Services Management: Implementation of the NHS Management Report (Griffiths Report), DHSS, London.

DHSS (1986) Report of the Community Nursing Review: Neighbourhood Nursing – A focus for care, HMSO, London.

DHSS (1988a) Report of the Inquiry into Child Abuse in Cleveland (Butler-Sloss) Cmnd 412, HMSO, London.

DHSS (1988b) Child Protection: guidance for senior nurses health visitors and midwives. Standing nursing and midwifery advisory committee (SNMAC), DHSS, London.

DHSS (1988c) Working Together: A guide to inter-agency cooperation for the protection of children from abuse, DHSS, London.

Dingwall, R., Eekelaar, J. and Murray, T. (1983) *The Protection of Children: state intervention in family life*, Basil Blackwell, Oxford.

Goodwin, S. (1988) Whither Health Visiting? *Health Visitor*, Dec., **61**(12), 379–383.

Goldblatt, P. (1988) Connections and adaptations, *Health Visitor*, Sept., **61**(9), 273–274.

Gough, P. and Hingley, P. (1988) Combating the pressure, *Nursing Times*, 13 Jan., **84**(2), 43–45.

HVA (1987) *A Stitch in Time: Perspectives on Management Structures for Health Visitors and School Nurses*, Health Visitors' Association, London.

London Borough of Brent (1985) A Child in Trust: The report of the panel of inquiry into the circumstances surrounding the death of Jasmine Beckford, London, London Borough of Brent.

London Borough of Greenwich (1987) A Child in Mind: Protection of children in a responsible society. The report of the commission of inquiry into the circumstances surrounding the death of Kimberley Carlile, London, London Borough of Greenwich.

McIntosh, J. and Dingwall, R. (eds) (1978) *Readings in the Sociology of Nursing*, Churchill Livingstone, Edinburgh.

Milne, D., Walker, L. and Bamford, S. (1987) Professional coping, *Health Visitor*, Feb., **60**, 49–50.

Ministry of Health (1966) Report of the Committee on Senior Nursing Staff Structure (Salmon Report), HMSO, London.

Munsen, C. E. (1976) Professional autonomy and social work supervision, *Journal of Education for Social Work*, Fall, **12**(3), 96–102.

Neuman, B. (1982) The Neuman Systems Model: Application to Nursing Education and Practice. Norwalk, Conn., Appleton Century Crofts.

Newberger, E. H. and Bourne, R. (1977) The medicalisation and legalisation of child abuse, in Eekelaar, J. M. and Katz (eds), *Family Violence: An international and interdisciplinary study*, Butterworths.

Parton, N. (1985) *The Politics of Child Abuse*, Macmillan, London.

Richardson, S. and Dunn, M. (1987) Coping with child abuse, Survival strategies for professionals, *Child Abuse Review*, Summer, **1**(6), 16.

Robinson, J. (1982) *An Evaluation of Health Visiting*, CETHV, London.

Smith, G. and Ames, J. (1976) Area teams in social work practice: A programme for research. *British Journal of Social Work*, **6**(1), 43–69.

Spicer, F. (1980) A support group for health visitors, *Health Visitor*, **53**(9), Sept., 377–379.

Vizard, E. (1983) Twenty months of Fridays – a support group for health visitors, *Health Visitor*, July, **56**, 255–256.

# CHAPTER TWELVE

# Occupational health nursing

## Marion Balcombe

A well recognized model of clinical supervision in occupational health nursing practice is hard to identify within the specialty, indeed, the question of whether one exists at all could well be asked. The nurse often works alone in an occupational health setting, and professional isolation presents its own problems—none more so than in the updating of skills and knowledge to maintain clinical credibility. The responsibility for this falls upon the individual who may not recognize the need.

In large organizations a number of people, with varying skills, may be employed within an occupational health unit, with the senior nurse, or possibly the occupational health physician, taking on the responsibility for clinical supervision. On occasion, however, this can lead to a narrow interpretation.

Regrettably, a qualification in the specialty is not a requirement for practice. It therefore follows that those nurses who have not undergone specialist training will have some difficulty in assessing their own level of practice. This difficulty is compounded by the lack of an organized framework of mentorship or supervision. The need for such is recognized, but the diversity of occupational health nursing practice brings with it its own constraints and only recently have some of these been addressed.

Before examining specific aspects surrounding the issue of clinical supervision, it is important that the reader has some knowledge of the background to occupational health nursing; the education and training available; the types of services offered, patterns of employment and variations in role. All of these have a bearing on present day models of care provided by the occupational health nurse.

History shows that 'industrial nurses' have been employed since 1878 (Charley, 1954). The First World War gave great impetus to the growing movement of caring for workers in the workplace. Regrettably, the forcing issue was a demand for shells rather than one of altruism. It was noted that fatigue inhibited production. A government report from 1915 quoted in Charley (1985) identifies that where nurses were in post, the health of the worker was seen to improve. The committee members were 'much impressed' as to the usefulness of competent nurses. Unhappily, post-war recession saw the depletion of industrial nursing services with many employers axing the service as an expensive luxury.

Developing ideas on prevention during the 1920s and 1930s involved some industrial nurses in embryonic health education programmes. It was soon realized by the most forward-thinking of them that the knowledge and skills they had acquired during their nurse training did not fit them for this emerging role. Members of the College of Nursing (now the RCN) campaigned for a specific course in industrial nursing. They were rewarded by the first course being set up in 1934.

The Second World War (1939–1945) again provided a stimulus for the provision of industrial nursing services and shortened courses of training were introduced. In 1950 collaboration between the International Labour Office and World Health Organizations (ILO–WHO) produced a report stating that 'occupational health should aim at the highest degree of physical, mental and social well-being of workers in all occupations'.

Shortly afterwards the RCN Industrial Nursing Certificate became the Occupational Health Nursing Certificate. Recent developments include the extension of the certificate programme to an academic year or equivalent; a modular concept for the six-weeks Occupational Practice Nurse Award; transfer of validation of both courses to the National Boards and emergence of diploma and degree programmes.

The geographical location and the number of courses available does not satisfy the need. The demand for courses, both full-time and part-time, is high. A major constraint for the full-time student, however, is lack of central funding. Health and Safety at work is currently the remit of the Department of Employment not the Department of Health. Occupational health nursing suffers considerably as a result of this and the majority of full-time students find that their only recourse is to self-fund. Day release students are, for the most part, sponsored by their employers.

Occupational health services are concerned with the effect of work on health, and the effect of health on the capacity to work. The type of service offered is dependent upon the interpretation of this definition. Some employers choose to see the implementation of the statutory first-aid service (Health and Safety (First Aid) Regulations 1981) as sufficient for their need. Others see the establishment of a nurse-orientated treatment service with the supplementary services of a part-time general practitioner, mainly concerned with pre-employment medical examinations, as the epitome of their development. A true occupational health service, however, provides a body of specialist knowledge, with specific objectives, i.e.

To assess, monitor and measure the working environment and advise on the necessary methods of control where hazard exists.

To be actively involved in the establishment of agreed health, safety and hygiene standards relevant to the particular establishments.

To assist management to utilise to best advantage the mental and physical abilities of those employed. (RCN, 1983)

Beyond this, an extended occupational health service may also include dentistry, physiotherapy, chiropody and other welfare facilities. Such services are, in the main, provided by large companies with qualified occupational health and safety practitioners (HSC, 1977). Additionally, the needs of small firms are increasingly being met by the provision of specialist advice from Group Occupational Services within both the public and private sectors.

The quality of care provided by an occupational service is dependent upon many factors, e.g. the type of service that management wishes to have and is able and willing to pay for; the specialist education and training of the staff involved; experience and personal motivation. Interfacing with all of these is the lack of a statutory requirement for the provision of occupational health services within the UK. This issue is compounded by the specialist qualification not being mandatory for practice. In consequence, services are variable and patchy.

There is no accurate information available on the exact number of nurses practising in occupational health in this country. Various estimates have been made. Radwanski (1982) suggested 9000, however, Dorward (1989) concludes from her research that 5000 would be a generous estimate. Exactly how many of these have specialist qualifications is again an unknown factor. Silverstone and Williams (1982) found that less than half of their respondents had undertaken any specialist training. This was an increase, however, on the previous research of Philips and McEwan (1979). Dorward (1989) found that 51.1% (i.e. 138 of her 270 respondents) had obtained the Occupational Health Nursing Certificate (open to first-level registered nurses only) and a further 22.2% had attended the Occupational Practice Award course or its predecessor the Part I course. Dorward concludes that there is an increasing trend for nurses to seek out specialist courses but availability is a major constraint.

An additional factor that must be considered is the number of nurses who have gained specialist qualifications who are no longer practising in occupational health. Around 3400 Occupational Health Nursing Certificates have been awarded since 1934. Research in 1983 (Balcombe, 1985) identified that 23% of certificate holders were no longer practising. This research concerned nurses who gained their certificate over the previous six years. It is disconcerting to reflect on the implications if this figure holds nationally.

Dorward's investigation reveals some interesting data, much of which is substantiated by previous research. The profile of the nurse who works in occupational health emerges as that of a mature woman, aged between 35–54 years, most likely to be a first-level nurse who first registered more than 10 years ago. She generally works alone; even if one of a number of nurses employed by a large organization, she is likely to be in sole charge of the occupational health unit while on duty. Many nurses are the only ones employed in the organization and will have received no particular preparation to work in occupational health. Their learning has taken place while in post, probably supplemented by attendance at a specialist course in occupational health nursing. The post she holds is quite likely to cover one industrial activity and be her first in occupational health. Her hours are full-time day duty only, with no weekend work.

While accepting that the majority of nurses employed in occupational health are industry-based, one must not forget the burgeoning occupational health services within the NHS, nor the areas of commerce and education where such services are increasingly developing. Indeed, many are well established.

All of the above factors have implications for professional practice, for the role of the nurse working in occupational health is one of great diversity. Complexity is added to diversity for the qualified occupational health nurse, i.e. the holder of the Occupational Health Nursing Certificate recordable on the single professional register of the UKCC. This certificate implies competence to practise over a wide range of activities, many of which range over the clinical spectrum.

The occupational health nurse is an independent practitioner with a professional advisory role in which confidentiality is paramount. She is responsible for her own actions and is ultimately accountable to the profession. Inevitably along with all other specialties, some elements of her nursing practice can be described as 'central core' while others are exclusive to the specialty (Turvey, 1984). In occupational health the extended role of the nurse takes on new meaning. This, for example, is recognized in statute The Medicines (Prescription Only) Amendment (No 2) Order 1978. This amendment to the Medicines Act of 1968 makes provision for occupational health nurses to administer Prescription Only medicines under a general written instruction signed by a doctor. This facility is further referred to in the UKCC advisory paper on the Administration of Medicines (1986) where it is recognized that dangerous delay could occur, with consequent risk to patients, if this facility were not available.

This is but one aspect of the extended role. When the full range of activities is considered other areas emerge. These may be examined under the previously mentioned headings of the effect of work on health or vice versa.

The RCN (1983) identified categories of activity with a view to enlightening prospective employers as to the potential in employing an occupational health nurse:

1.  *Effects of work on health*
    Monitoring of the environment and the development of control methods.
    Identification of advice on hazards.
    Periodic examination related to identified risk.
    Provision of emergency care for casualties.
    Interpretation of the law, i.e. factory, commercial, professional.
    Health supervision of welfare facilities, e.g. canteen.
    Health education/health advice.
    Epidemiological studies, sickness absence.
    Disaster planning.
2.  *Effects of health on work*
    Examination relative to job demands, e.g. pre-employment, special hazards.
    Assessment of capacity after sickness and advice on fitness for task; rehabilitation and resettlement.
    Care of special groups, e.g. disabled, young, pregnant.
    Health advice to employees/clients.

From within this framework a diverse and potentially demanding role emerges. This role is catered for within the outline curriculum of the certificate programme which covers the following areas: health supervision in the workplace, health education and health promotion, communication skills, general and specific environmental monitoring, occupational health and safety, toxicity, accident prevention, relevant legislation, organization of emergency treatment services for accidents and illness arising at work, rehabilitation, outside agencies and support services, first-aid training, administration/record-keeping/report-writing, research activities.

Extrapolating areas from these curricula that could be defined as 'clinical' is not as easy as it would first appear. Much depends on the accepted definition of 'clinical'. The Concise Oxford Dictionary defines clinical as 'of or at the sick bed', a definition virtually useless in terms of occupational health nursing practice. A more acceptable definition, located in 'Words' (1956), is 'based on actual observation: not theoretical'. This would seem to link comfortably with the philosophy expressed by the editors in the introduction to this book—namely the belief that nurses have much to learn from each other. (It is interesting to note that a description from 1956 remains so apt in 1991.)

Before developing this further in the context of occupational health, the more obvious clinical aspects of the specialty and the nurse's role within them will be explored.

## Treatment services

The pros and cons of providing a treatment service within an occupational health service have been discussed many times. There are those who believe quite passionately that routine treatments should never be included and that the service should be seen to be entirely preventative in approach. Indeed, in France, treatment is expressly forbidden although unofficially some choose to ignore this. Similarly, a Department of Health advisory circular (1982) on the setting up of occupational health services within the NHS does not give consideration to a treatment service being offered but again this is often ignored. The protagonists of treatment services suggest that it is in the therapeutic role that reputations are made and confidence inspired. This leads on more readily to acceptance of the preventive, promotive role. Essentially, many managements view a treatment service as providing cost benefits while some practitioners would argue that this is an incorrect use of service resources (Taylor and Ward-Gardner, 1981). Interestingly, treatment services were actively discouraged in the ILO recommendations No. 112 (1959). However, the recent revision (1985) which also produced Convention No. 161 and Recommendation No. 171 re-introduces treatment as a recognized and necessary component within some occupational health services.

Whichever view one is inclined to, the fact remains that the majority of occupational health nurses are involved in the dispensation of treatment to a greater or lesser extent. Silverstone and Williams (1982) identified 86% of nurses involved in 'care of the injured and sick' to some degree. The author's own research in 1983 supported this finding with 18% of the occupational health nurses' time being involved with treatment.

The focus of this must be centred on the fact that occupational health nurses have no automatic authority to treat. Clinically, as far as treatment is concerned, they are accountable to an occupational health physician where one is employed: few such are full time within an organization, but those who are usually hold a specialist qualification. The majority are part-time general practitioners without specialist training (Select Committee, 1983).

In all traditional clinical procedures the nurse has a responsibility to maintain standards. In the hospital situation, there is constant analysis and reinforcement of techniques, often established and evaluated in a team setting. The team provides a focus of support and a dynamic model of care evolves. This scenario exists in occupational health within well established teams but for many nurses who work alone clinical practice may become out of date without realizing it. Interestingly, Dorward found the acquisition of 'further clinical skills' an important element in reasons for attending courses.

The question of indemnity insurance is an important one in occupational health where nurses may be asked to carry out clinical procedures that traditionally have not been seen as part of the nurse's role, e.g. ear-syringing. The nurse must be satisfied as to her own competence and work within an agreed, written, local operational policy. Even then difficulties may arise when what is seemingly a simple nursing procedure becomes questionable because of the circumstances in which it is to be carried out. Turvey (1984) cites as an example a procedure such as a desensitizing injection, simple in nursing terms, but quite inappropriate if risks of anaphylaxis exist and suitable support expertise and equipment do not. Refusal to carry out the procedure may be misunderstood by both employers and employees who may not understand the risks involved. A high level of interpersonal skill is often required to countermand a potentially explosive situation. Indeed, interpersonal skills are constantly brought into play within all the activities of an occupational health service and none more so than with the reluctant patient. Reluctant, that is, to accept that all is not well and a second immediate opinion is called for. Classic here is the stoical middle-aged man presenting with 'indigestion' but wanting to get back to work as quickly as possible; time often means money in this situation. Clinical judgement assumes a more serious condition. The lone nurse needs to have total confidence in her assessment as her advisory role becomes persuasive. Indeed, her reputation may well stand or fall on the outcome of just such a situation. Emphasis must lie heavily on the 'lone nurse' who operates effectively without supervision. The responsibility for a decision made rests entirely with her.

## Health supervision and screening

The exercise of clinical judgement frequently extends beyond treatment into the remit of diagnosis and referral. Health supervision and screening programmes demand a high level of expertise which can become endangered by repetition. A vast amount of nursing time may be involved in the screening of apparently fit and healthy personnel. The nurse needs to be constantly alert to the possibility of error in both judgement and technique. This becomes doubly important when working alone without the stimulus of colleagues.

Ongoing assessment of those individuals and groups at special risk involves the nurse in much more than purely clinical assessment of the person; the environment in which they work is equally of importance. The nursing process becomes a familiar tool as planning, implementation and evaluation follow ongoing assessment and become part of the rhythm of daily routine.

### Counselling

Counselling is a concept fraught with ambiguity. It means different things to different people, and therefore the assessment of how much time the occupational health nurse spends in a counselling situation is open to argument. Many nurses feel that much of their work is taken up with counselling activities. However, Williams (1981) found that only 5% of an occupational health nurse's time was devoted to counselling. The authors own research (Balcombe, 1983) established 7% of time spent on counselling and health advice. Clearly there is a difference between perceived and actual time spent but undoubtedly it is a 'preferred' activity with which nurses wish to become more familiar.

It is also an activity that can create anxiety and the occupational health nurse is no less vulnerable than other carers in this respect. Indeed, her isolation may increase vulnerability and the need for a support system. Training and experiential learning is a critical factor in the nurse's ability to cope satisfactorily with the art of counselling. If a client becomes overly dependent, the result can be disastrous for both client and nurse. Confidentiality can be eroded unintentionally as stress levels rise and this should be precluded by early referral; often the optimum time for this is missed due to lack of training. The occupational health nurse's anxiety over counselling is substantiated in Dorward's study where counselling emerges as a priority in continuing education needs.

Having identified several areas of the nurse's role, normally acceptable as 'clinical practice', the supervisory relationship relative to the terms of this book may be examined.

### Supervision and mentorship

If 'clinical supervision is an enabling relationship between nurses whereby one nurse is accountable to another nurse in helping them practise to the best of their ability', then a variety of models emerge within the specialty. Their application is dependent upon source and location. Although the number of qualified occupational health nurses is increasing, a considerable number are practising without a specialist qualification; this accounts to some degree for fluctuation in standards. Additionally, many are enrolled nurses who are eligible for the Practice Nurse Award only.

Whilst on a course the traditional teacher/pupil model of supervision predominates. On part-time courses the course tutor will normally visit the student in her place of work where various activities will be observed. Such visits are, however, infrequent, and the student needs support from other sources. This may well be provided by fellow students on the days in college. The value of such contact is undisputed but again there are limiting factors. The perceived need of alternative support for day-release students has been met in some instances by the instigation of a mentorship scheme. A qualified occupational health nurse from an organization local to the student takes on this responsibility in a supportive but non-judgemental role. The student may visit for periods of alternative practice experience as well as having support in particular problem areas.

This mentorship scheme differs from the 'practical placement' allocation of a full-time student. Here the 'supervisor', usually qualified and experienced in occupational health, is expected to provide a facilitative learning environment and report on the student's ability to work within it.

Unlike other community specialties, until recently there has been little provision for the training of practical placement supervisors. One or two colleges only are providing 'facilitator' programmes of between one and three days. However, the advent of the ENB community practice teacher course may well correct this anomaly, although it is recognized that funding may prove difficult. Additionally, this course allows for the development of a period of supervised practice as a requirement for qualification and the award of the Occupational Health Nursing Certificate. Occupational health nurse teachers have long recognized such a need, especially with regard to full-time students with no previous experience in occupational health. Additionally, refresher and updating programmes should be ongoing. The occupational health nurse has an individual professional responsibility to maintain competence.

In this context, the nurse operating within a team as part of a national or multi-national organization is in a very different position from the lone occupational health nurse in a medium-sized or small company. The large organization with structured occupational health services frequently arranges for 'in-house' courses thus enabling their nurses to be kept up to date, new principles to be established, and the possibility of practice-induced stress to be reduced.

## OCCUPATIONAL HEALTH SERVICE

Having said earlier that there is no one model of clinical supervision that is generic to occupational health nursing, it is important to identify a mode of good practice that lends itself to adaptation. The following is an example of how a truly preventive occupational health service can be integrated with a treatment service where there is specific need for the latter. The organization in question is a large company involved in food production.

The occupational health service is headed by the Group Occupational Health Adviser—a qualified and very experienced occupational health nurse with a diverse background of professional and management experience. She reports to the Personnel Director. Her staff consists of 12 occupational health nursing officers, all of whom are experienced and qualified in the specialty; all are peripatetic. Additionally, there are six static nurses who provide a treatment service in high-risk situations, e.g. a site with 600–1000 employees where the process involves the use of knives. The static nurse may be an RGN or EN. All the nurses work to well-defined written policies, procedures and standards which they are expected to interpret in a way that allows for professional discretion. They have a functional accountability to the Group Occupational Health Adviser on all professional matters; administratively they report to the individual site managers, with whom they are expected to debate and negotiate on the implementation of policies and maintenance of standards.

The occupational health service manual is compiled and regularly updated by the Group Occupational Health Adviser; it is widely available within the organization. The content is clearly defined under five headings:

1. Occupational Health Service
   - policy
   - objectives
   - roles of occupational health personnel
   - procedures
2. Fitness Standards
3. Guidelines: Prevention
4. Occupational Health Service Staff
   - procedures
   - information
5. First Aid

The health and safety policy identifies the company's responsibilities under the Health and Safety at Work Act 1974 and extends this to include moral and economic considerations.

The occupational health policy follows accepted principles, stressing its advisory function and emphasizing that:

> it is complementary to the NHS, providing facilities at the workplace not otherwise available; the service should not interfere with the relationship between the employee and the family doctor.

The objectives of the service identify the Group Occupational Health Adviser's role. It is clear that within the new broader concept of clinical supervision this role is extended. It includes the professional development of her staff and the ensuring of professional standards by offering advice and support where necessary.

The occupational health officers have wide-ranging responsibilities concerned with the prevention of ill health, the promotion of positive health and concepts of safety. Their involvement in health supervision, examination and screening, allows for referral to a medical practitioner only when necessary. Such referral consists of medical examination by a 'location medical officer'. These are usually retained general practitioners employed for their clinical skills only on an 'item of service' payment. The examination usually takes place in the general practitioner's surgery and is conducted to laid-down procedures within the manual.

In any nurse or doctor recommendation as to 'fitness' or 'unfitness' for employment, confidentiality is paramount. The certificate should simply state 'fit' with restrictions, or 'unfit' for work without any mention of medical details.

The confidentiality of 'medical' records is one which may be frequently challenged. All doubt as to confidentiality is allayed within this organization by the procedures laid down for the retention of the access to occupational health records. If a management investigation leads to a request for the disclosure of occupational health/medical information, this is channelled through the Occupational Health Adviser. She informs the occupational health officer who establishes whether the records identify any relevant information; if so, only this fact is relayed to management who then have the responsibility of obtaining the written consent of the employee for the release of relevant data.

The rest of the occupational health manual is concerned with general and specific fitness standards, the implementation of preventive techniques and information on procedures to ensure a degree of standardization of measurement and recording. All of these align to the general principles of maintaining professional nursing standards, some of which relate to defined competencies, while others are more facilitative. This service is nurse-led and therefore departs from the medical model that is still widely seen. Despite the fact that the Faculty of Occupational

Medicine, within the Royal College of Physicians, agreed some years ago that where a nurse is qualified and full-time and the doctor is part-time, the nurse should head the service, this is frequently not so. Nevertheless, the nurse-orientated service is gaining ground with access to medical practitioners as required.

Within the service as described, the nurses receive the education, training, advice and support that they need. The occupational health officers are autonomous practitioners operating within defined areas of accountability. Many lone nurses within small organizations are denied such facilities and need to develop initiatives that will ensure acceptable professional standards. The peer group support often experienced within groups of students is further developed once a course has ended: a network of information can result and a mutual 'counselling' service emerges. Beyond this, many occupational health nurses attend specialist group meetings, study days and refresher courses. Many large companies now invite nurses from outside their organization to their internal courses and this becomes mutually beneficial.

Additionally some occupational health teachers operate 'associate programmes' integrated with the certificate programme on a sessional basis. These programmes allow for the attendance of both qualified and unqualified nurses and serve as very useful refresher courses.

A further source of support is the Employment Medical Advisory Service (EMAS). This is the operative arm of the Medical Division of the Health and Safety Executive. Within this organization, there is a national regional network of Employment Nursing Advisers who are ready to assist any occupational health nurse who seeks their advice.

The Royal College of Nursing continues to be a source of support and information through its Society of Occupational Health Nursing and its Professional Adviser. Additionally, the Occupational Health Nurse Managers' Forum, within the Association of Nursing Management, provides valuable updating via their one-day conferences.

Increasingly, in this commercial world, pharmaceutical supply companies sponsor study days whilst advertising their new and existing products. This is a valuable service providing updating for nurses in clinical products and much discussion between those who have tried them.

The Occupational Health Committee of the English National Board for Nursing, Midwifery and Health Visiting monitors educational standards while the specialist education officers are frequently called upon for professional support and advice.

Incredibly, although occupational health nursing has been a reality for so many years, it is only now emerging as a specialty deserving of recognition by the UKCC. The certificate has become a recordable qualification; the role is encompassed within that of the specialist practitioner in health promotion under the auspices of Project 2000—a new preparation for practice. What exactly this will entail is, as yet, undecided.

## REFERENCES

Balcombe, M. (1985) Image and reality, *Occupational Health*, **37**, 5–7.

Chadsey, P., Morris, W. and Wentworth, H. (1956) *Words – the New Illustrated Dictionary*, Spring Books, London.

Charley, I. H. (1954) *The Birth of Industrial Nursing*, Baillière Tindall, London (Reprinted 1978).

Department of Health and Social Security, Health Notice (82)33, *Health Services Management OH Services for NHS Staff*, HMSO.

Dorward, A. L. (1989) *Continuing Education Needs of Nurses Working in Occupational Health*, HSE Research Paper 27, HMSO.

Health and Safety (First Aid) Regulations (1981) HMSO.

Health and Safety Commission (1977) *Occupational Health Service: The Way Ahead*, HMSO, London.

I.L.O. Occupational Health Services Convention (1985) HMSO.

Philips, M. and McEwan, J. J. (1979) Private occupational health services in Britain, The EMAS Survey, 1976, Department of Community Health, University of Nottingham.

Radwanski, D. (1982) The forgotten nine thousand, *Nursing Mirror*, 155/14, 46–47.

Royal College of Nursing (1983) (reprinted 1987) *A Handbook for Employers and Nurses*, Society of OH Nursing.

Select Committee on Science and Technology: House of Lords (1983) *Occupational Health and Hygiene Services*, Vol. 1, HMSO.

Silverstone, R. and Williams, A. (1982) *The role and educational needs of occupational health nurses*, RCN.

Taylor, P. J. and Ward Gardner (1981) *Treatment and First-Aid Services in Occupational Health Practice* (3rd edition), Butterworth, 1989.

Turvey, K. (1984) *Clinical Standards in Occupational Health Nursing*, supplement to *Nursing*, 2nd series, Medical Education International Limited.

Williams, M. M. D. (1981) *Counselling in Occupational Health Nursing*, RCN.

# CHAPTER THIRTEEN

# District nursing

## *Brian Pateman*

### INTRODUCTION

This chapter is an overview discussing some of the factors that promote good practice in district nursing. It begins with a short history of district nursing to give some insight to those readers who are unfamiliar with it. This is important as it locates district nursing within the particular influences that have helped to shape and give it a particular ideological position.

Education and training for district nurses is discussed; this will be of particular interest to those with no experience of community nursing, given the present development of mentorship schemes in general nurse education, as the use of a practical work teacher and supervisor in the clinical setting is a long established practice in district nursing. Literature on post-qualification supervision and good practice in district nursing is hard to find. This chapter reports on an opinion survey carried out among senior nurses and practising district nurses in the Greater Manchester area, in an attempt to find out opinions and action strategies from the field.

There are a number of related matters which impinge on the general area of supervision. Quality assurance which shows some promise in the raising of standards is not discussed in any great depth although reference will be made to it. There is a wealth of information on the subject elsewhere, so much so that it requires at least a chapter on its own.

Finally, self-evaluation and peer review is promoted as a method of achieving good practice via peer supervision. Although it is used by many nurses at an informal level at the moment, this model needs more formalization in order to maximize its potential.

## DEVELOPMENT OF DISTRICT NURSING

Nursing has had some history of basing clinical expertise on tasks and procedures, rather than on sound theoretical principles. Good practice has been measured by the speed and efficiency with which a nurse could discharge her allotted tasks. Nursing is now carried out in more enlightened times. There is much talk of 'individualized care, primary nursing, team nursing and patient allocation' with the result that 'task' allocation is becoming an outmoded concept. How has district nursing been affected by changes occurring in the views of mainstream nursing as to what constitutes good practice and how far have these new ideas been included in practice?

District nursing has always been seen as a post-registration experience and therefore this has led many to conceptualize community nursing in terms of hospital experience when explaining their role to student nurses. 'I am like a ward sister whose ward stretches from the gas works to the market; I am assisted by an Enrolled Nurse and an Auxiliary; our doctor is the local GP.' It is apparent that some of the concepts, principles, values and management structure to be found in present-day district nursing have an institutional origin. It has not always been so.

The greatest influence on standards in district nursing in its infancy was the Queen's Nursing Institute (QNI), which can trace its origins back to 1887. The QNI was responsible for training and monitoring standards in district nursing before state registration started with the setting up of the General Nursing Council in 1919.

QNI training was often task-focused and procedural. There were inflexible rules to follow when performing procedures such as bed bathing, dressing wounds, injections, etc. The training was seen to be of a high standard and led to the development of good standards of practice in the community. Often improvisation was essential; nurses were faced with the problem of attempting to deliver high quality nursing care totally unsupported by materials which modern district nursing takes for granted, such as social services and pre-packed sterile dressings and instruments. Procedures in the patient's home were carried out with what the nurse could either carry herself or borrow from the patient. Chairs became backrests, biscuit tins when placed in ovens became autoclaves to sterilize the dressings and instruments were boiled in pans. Queen's nurses will often recall being taught how to fold old newspaper to make disposal bags. Despite this 'Heath Robinson' approach, high standards of technical competence were ensured that could be measured by district nurse supervisors.

All that the supervisors of district nurses had to do was to check that procedures being performed conformed to the strict procedural instructions from the QNI. It is important to note however that a distinct 'district nurse' culture was fostered by the QNI and part of that culture was the notion of proper supervision of individualized practice.

District nursing, although developing from hospital-based practice, differed from hospital nursing in that individualized care could always be practised due to the very nature of the one-to-one relationship.

District nursing in those early days consisted of much more than technical skills; the nurse worked as social worker, home help, health visitor and nurse, but these additional skills were often learnt by experience, maturity and 'sitting by Nellie' rather than from a formal curriculum. The training consisted of task orientation and a hidden 'social skills' curriculum that was learned informally. There have been times however when district nursing was seen in less than glowing terms. In 1953 a government working party was set up to look at care in the community. They received very strong representation from doctors, social workers and health visitors. District nurses, assuming that their worth would be automatically recognized, did not feel the need to give an account of themselves as other community-based professionals had done. As a result the 1955 Report of the Working Party on the Training of District Nurses came as a shock. Instead of recommending an increase, as was widely expected, in the length of district nurse training to take account of their developing role, the suggestion was made that it could be shortened. This suggestion was made on an assumption that because of improved social conditions in the community, training for district nurses could be reduced, whilst other group training was to be extended! Low morale amongst district nurses resulted from the report with a general feeling that they had been 'sold down the river'.

In more recent times greater value has been placed on district nursing. Since 1981 training has been mandatory for nurses wishing to practise as DNs and linked with higher education. Their training takes nine months split into two distinct parts: taught practice and supervised practice. There is six months of taught practice of which two-thirds is clinical practice with a Practical Work Teacher (PWT) and one-third theory conducted in a university or polytechnic. The final three months is a period of supervised practice.

## SUPERVISION IN THE EDUCATION OF DISTRICT NURSES

### Taught practice with a community practice teacher (CPT)

The CPT is an experienced district nurse who can demonstrate good practice in her/his work and will have undertaken the CPT course. This equips the CPT with the necessary teaching, assessment and counselling skills that are necessary for teaching a student district nurse. In most cases the CPT functions as a normal district nurse with a caseload. In 1987 CPTs were awarded grade H on the salary scale, in recognition of their extra workload and responsibility.

During their four months of practical training the students practise under the close instruction and supervision of a CPT and progress through stages similar to those outlined by Benner (1984):

1. observer/novice;
2. practice under direct supervision/advanced beginner;
3. practice under remote supervision/competent;
4. proficiency.

Proficiency is the last stage achieved in district nursing under supervised practice. Having successfully completed the taught practice element of training the student then proceeds to supervised practice when they have responsibility for a full but controlled caseload for three months. The supervisor is a different experienced DN who has undertaken a supervisors' course and acts as an adviser and supporter rather than a teacher. As well as this mentorship role the supervisor has an important role to play in monitoring standards, ensuring that the basic competencies are satisfied and promoting higher order good practice over and above the minimum.

## The CPT–student relationship

One might reasonably expect the relationship between the CPT and the student to be one of superior teacher and dependent student. In practice this is not the case and the relationship is more one of a partnership, with the CPT acting as a mentor and facilitator rather than as an authoritarian figure. Student and CPT work together to negotiate training needs, as many students will have considerable post-registration experience which needs to be taken into account when planning student programmes. It is often the case that students will have particular skills or knowledge which the DN team can draw upon. The overall aim is to maximize the students' abilities by drawing on their past experiences. The process of education will continue even if minimum requirements are satisfied early. The student is encouraged and supported to maximize their potential.

John Dobby (1981) carried out research for the DHSS evaluating the procedures used to assess the practical work of DN students. The questions to be asked and ideas to be explored included:

1. Do assessment procedures make unrealistic demands on those carrying it out (the CPT)?

2. What consensus of student grading existed between the various education centres? This was required for monitoring and to justify the course as a qualification with a national standard.
3. To highlight any inadequacies in the system and formulate suggestions for improvement.
4. As training post-1981 would be mandatory there was a need to develop an effective assessment tool to judge the skills and attributes of potential students thus minimizing wastage in DN training.

In this study practical assessment forms from all the centres were collated and analysed in an attempt to find common criteria. There was evidence of considerable disagreement between centres on the qualities a DN should possess. The aggregate criteria of items to be assessed came to 500 headings, which was an indication of how complex assessing district nursing is or how widely the role of the district nurse was interpreted by the various centres.

The shortcomings of using criteria for assessment based on tasks and inflexible procedures rather than on principles were highlighted by this work. The following example is given by Dobby (1981). Nurse X is much better than nurse Y at using voluntary services. Analysis of this statement shows that it is ambiguous. The question to ask is how predictive is a behavioural objective at determining behaviour; for example Nurse Y may have a greater knowledge but lacks the opportunity to demonstrate that knowledge.

This study found much evidence pointing to generalization without discrimination. This could be seen in assessments where poor and good candidates had all their marks in the respective poor or good rating columns. There was also considerable variation in grading student performance.

Dobby suggested a peripatetic CPT, senior nurse or tutor to moderate the assessment of students which would also reduce the stress of assesment and improve validity. In practice this suggestion has been found to be unworkable although those CPTs who team teach are in an excellent position to compare and contrast students.

One assessment form received particular praise by Dobby as it made clinical practice as important as formative assessment. On this particular form it was necessary to record student weakness and the action taken. This diagnostic and prescriptive approach has much to merit it even though it focused on negative rather than positive strengths. DN students are now assessed continuously using formative assessment to develop potential as far above the minimum competencies as is possible. The self-assessment element encourages students to continue to develop their own development rather than training being seen as once and for all.

One of the problems of the role model approach to training by attaching a student closely to an experienced practitioner is that it might produce mirror images of that practitioner, with all her/his weaknesses as well as her/his strengths. Supervised practice helps to minimize this as students have a different supervisor/mentor and usually change working areas so they are confronted with new philosophies and working practices which will differ from those they may have already encountered.

## POST-QUALIFICATION—CLINICAL SUPERVISION PROMOTING GOOD PRACTICE

### Senior nurse's role

Understandably much is made of promoting good practice and supervision during training. However there is less information relating to the supervision of trained DNs, apart from the emerging literature on quality assurance, quality circles and tools such as monitor.

In an attempt to discover what was being done in the practice setting the author surveyed 11 senior nurses (district nursing) in the Greater Manchester area and asked questions about the methods they saw as promoting good practice. There was a wide diversity of opinion. Senior nurses quite clearly had radically differing opinions. It was evident that there were pressing financial concerns at the time of the survey which were very much at the forefront of any discussions.

*Quality Assurance.* Eight of the 11 senior nurses contacted mentioned quality assurance as a method of promoting good practice. Two who were in the early stages of implementation were most optimistic; of the other six four were quite advanced, having set performance criteria in pilot areas. Three were unsure and the other three were having doubts based on the time-consuming nature of the exercise. One stated that there were many 'spin-offs' leading to improvements in targeting service provision following a consumer survey linked to the quality assurance programme: a human 'MOT' clinic and a leg ulcer clinic were examples given.

Many saw the process as useful but were put off by how long it was all taking. There was evidence of disagreement about the usefulness of multidisciplinary review. One senior nurse was most adamant that other professionals, especially GPs, had insufficient fine detail of the DN role to be able to comment. However most took the view (most notably those involved in well-advanced quality assurance programmes) that multidisciplinary review is essential as all workers rely on each other even if it is just to receive referrals. This demonstrates a variable view that nurses have about opening up their work to wider multidisciplinary review.

*Supervision of Practice.* 'Supervision rounds', where a senior nurse visits patients with the district nurse, was mentioned by all the senior nurses. One thought of them as not being useful as situations could be manipulated, patients could be primed and the presence of a senior nurse could hamper performance. However, although the majority felt it to be a highly beneficial strategy it was considered to be too time consuming and therefore too difficult to be used regularly. The senior nurse has to be selective in using this strategy but as Baly (1981) noted, a good indication of the standard of care can be obtained:

> another nurse visiting a patient will inevitably notice the standard of care by observing the availability of equipment, the plans of care, the involvement and attitude of patient and other carers.

One senior nurse saw directly observed clinical supervision as a most effective tool in encouraging, monitoring and maintaining standards of care. She defended the time commitment involved in the exercise by saying that it facilitated senior nurses to function in their real role as supervisors and monitors of good quality services.

*In-Service Training.* All senior nurses stated a commitment to in-service training for new techniques and products. Some areas had been more reluctant than usual to send nurses on courses that could be interpreted as role extension or specialization because it may lead to claims for a higher salary grade, particularly if they are to cascade or network the information to peers upon return. It is ironic that a salary grade implemented to develop clinical expertise may be having just the opposite effect.

*Nursing Process.* One respondent mentioned examining the nursing process notes as a good method of evaluating the care given. The Open University package 'A Systematic Approach to Nursing Care' was found to be useful by many not only to improve care plans but nursing practice as well. In a similar way nursing models were seen as a tool to reflect upon nursing practice.

*Peer Review.* When questioned about peer and case review the senior nurses stated that there was no formal implementation of these practices but, informally, DNs discussed and evaluated each other's practice. Peer support occurs naturally as Baly (1981) observed, however, this is not always as proactive and dynamic as it could be.

*Peer Support.* There were many examples of peer support, information and ideas sharing in day-to-day work. One particular group of nurses
changed caseloads and visited each other's patients on a frequent ad hoc
basis. All nurses stated the value of colleagues from their own team and
others who visited their patients on days off, etc., who were able to make
suggestions or be positively critical.

*Skill Mix.* An acting director of nursing services states a most
interesting example of promoting good practice, whereby a part-time
health visitor was replaced by a secretary at the request of the health
visitors on a trial basis. Not only did the standard of note keeping and
letter writing improve, but the health visitors were less harassed as they
no longer had to complete records out of hours at home. They also felt
that their status had improved. This is an example of how skill mix can
effect morale and practice and an indication that support workers need
not be auxiliary nurses under another name.

## Specialist nurses in the community

One of the anticipated areas of excellence in the community would be
specialist nurses who act as experts in a particular field and therefore
would be expected to develop good practice within the narrower
parameters of their boundaries. There are mixed feelings over these posts
amongst DNs; some welcome colleagues who can improve the quality of
care via their superior knowledge and resources, others see it as
devaluation and dissipation of the role of the DN as an expert generalist.
Cannam and Murray (1989) have expressed a wish to see DNs trained in
a specialty so that each DN will have a specialist interest in addition to
their 'traditional' role. However, this might precipitate problems when
general workloads become heavy and consequently specialist commitments receive low priority. There is a prevailing view that specialist
nurses have best value when, instead of developing a separate caseload in
isolation from mainstream district nurses, they work as specialist advisers
to, and work with those district nurses.

## Nurse managers' role in promoting good practice

The Griffiths review of the NHS has led to the imposition of a more
businesslike control of the services. The 'buzz' words of the late 1980s
and 1990s seems to be quality, cost effectiveness and performance.
Quality assurance is seen by many in management to hold the key to
good practice. However, as Hallett (1989) has pointed out:

The heart of good quality is not technique but commitment by management to its people and patients it serves along with knowledgeable management practice.

She goes on to say, 'There is a danger that the quality assurance train will run out of steam if superficial and simplistic interventions are implemented. Good practice will not originate from discussions taking place at conferences but from good management of staff, resources and promoting good standards of care.'

One obstacle that stands in the way of developing innovative new practices is that nurses see the needs of their existing patients as having a higher priority over investing in new strategies for the future. There is reluctance in spending time on a quality circle when a patient needs attention.

Hallett ends her article by voicing a concern that 'Indicators are beginning to appear which point to the imposition of non-nursing managers taking responsibility for nursing departments'. This will surely hamper the cause of good clinical practice if, as stated earlier, good practice depends not on technique but on the commitment of all involved in the system. It follows that this requires nursing knowledge to argue the case for good practice rather than just good accountancy. Problems of this sort have been reported in the press; for example, in the district nursing service at Oldham, external consultants carried out an evaluation of the district nursing service in which they concluded that much greater productivity could be achieved in the service by stopping the nurses talking to the patients so that more tasks could be performed by each nurse.

## Autonomy/accountability and management

There has been an increasing move towards autonomous nursing practice in the community, and as a consequence, district nurses are becoming more accountable for their actions. Through the implementation of the Griffiths Report, decision making, budgets and accountability are moving ever closer to those who have to deliver the service.

As practice nurses develop new skills, district nurses argue about extended roles. This is not a new argument. Hockey (1978) asked the rhetorical question: 'First visits by nurses to patients who have asked a doctor to call. Is this a new role suitable for a nurse or not?' She then proceeds to answer her own question:

I believe it is a retrograde step to make a rule by creating a role. The professionals, Doctor and Nurses should come to a mutually acceptable agreement in the light of the individual patient and the situation.

Too many rules not only hamper autonomy and accountability but also reduce the required flexibility to answer new demands.

One health authority in the Mersey Region has an interesting approach to district nurse management. Senior nurses who are given the title coordinators are all clinical nurses with a reduced patient caseload and therefore can be seen to be fully in touch with the clinical area.

This system has potential for promoting overt rather than covert good practice. Taking rehabilitation as an example, a lack of accident reports and evidence of a clean and tidy patient could be taken as good nursing practice by a remote management, although the opposite could be true and the patient might well have lost all autonomy and be dependent on others for all activities of daily living. Clinical supervision by nurses with an active, recent clinical knowledge will help to focus on a more accurate account of nurse intervention.

## Peer support and evaluation

Increasing autonomy, accountability and self-determination can cause stress, while management support is essential and peer support can form a vital base for practice. Bond (1982) discussed types of peer support to relieve stress. Like the nursing process many nurses may say peer support is carried out already, but they have not conceptualized or analysed the process. As district nurses practise on their own it is essential that they seek the support of their peers through their opinions and advice.

*Direct support.* Loyalty and an approachable attitude are essential attributes within the nursing team to create a supporting atmosphere so that good practice can be achieved through a willingness to share advice and seek help.

*Practical help.* District nurses often assist each other by sharing a workload, but this is dependent on the nurse being assertive enough to admit to needing help. This can be construed as evidence, real or imagined, of incompetence and failure to manage. On the other hand it also depends on the helper declaring that they have sufficient time to help.

*Sharing information.* The independent nature of the district nursing work means that information sharing is essential. Some district nurses have journal clubs. CPTs in some areas share not only information but team teach their students.

*Sharing problems.* It is essential for district nurses to seek help from peers with problems in order that the best solution within known constraints is obtained.

Discussion over action to be taken could take several forms:

1. Acting as a sounding board allowing the person to come to their own conclusion as to the best course of action.
2. Offering suggestions for action.
3. Encouraging and supporting colleagues by agreeing:
   a) that the action decided upon is appropriate, or
   b) that perfection may not be readily attainable and this action is the best one within poor circumstances.
4. Learning through others' triumphs and failures.

Discussion of problems must be constructive and not critical. The idea being to help not attack, comments such as: 'You should've' or 'You've got to' or 'I always' are neither helpful nor tactful. It is important for both advice giver and receiver to realize that advice does not have to be taken.

*Role playing, hypothetical case discussion.* Rehearsal of difficult situations, i.e. bereavement and ethical problems can be practised to aid decision making in actual situations.

*Peer evaluation.* As stated earlier, peer review occurs whether it is formalized into work practices or not. Peer evaluation can be a most effective tool in raising good practice if elevated to constructive feedback. To be effective it needs courage and trust and the realization that it is the practice and not the person who is being reviewed. Criticism needs to be balanced with praise. There needs to be the courage to give and receive constructive criticism taking care to prevent the imposition of one's own standards, beliefs and work practices upon others.

## REFERENCES

Baly, M. (Ed.) (1981) *A New Approach To District Nursing*, Heinemann, London.
Benner, P. (1984) *From Novice to Expert*, Addison-Wesley, London.
Bond, M. (1982) *Stress and Self Awareness – A Guide For Nurses*, Heinemann, London.
Cannam, J. and Murray, C. (1989) The community specialist, *Journal of District Nursing*, December, 10–12.

Caring for Patients (1989) (Government White Paper on the NHS) HMSO, London.

Caring for People (1989) *Community Care in the Next Decade and Beyond* (Government White Paper, Replying to the 'Griffiths' report on community care), HMSO, London.

Dobby, J. (1981) *An Evaluation of the Procedures used to Assess the Practical Work of District Nurse Trainees*, Brunel University, Research for DHSS.

Hallett, S. (1989) Managing for quality, *Senior Nurse*, 9(7), July.

Hockey (1978) The future nurse: Selection and training; autonomy; should her health care role be modified for future patient demands, *Journal of Advanced Nursing*, 3, 571–582.

Open University (1984) *P553 A Systematic Approach To Nursing Care: An Introduction*, The Open University Press, Milton Keynes.

# CHAPTER FOURTEEN

# Clinical supervision in community psychiatric nursing

*Peter Wilkin*

By the early 1980s research into community psychiatric nursing was beginning to highlight a need for a more theoretically-based, universal approach to community care, flexible enough to accommodate a variety of therapeutic interventions. As yet, the search for such an approach has proved difficult, the main stumbling blocks being the variety of skills employed by Community Psychiatric Nurses (CPNs), further complicated by the wide range of mental health problems which they encounter. How can a model of nursing, which a psychodynamically-orientated CPN is using to treat someone with a marital problem, be used just as effectively by a CPN with behavioural skills whose client is complaining of adverse side-effects from his depot injection? What is needed is a common language to describe practice, recognizable by all CPNs, no matter which way they choose to work. The intention of this chapter is to propose a model of supervision, which can provide a theoretical base to underpin all CPN interventions and also be utilized as a resource for evaluating action.

Supervision is a dynamic, interpersonally focused experience which promotes the development of therapeutic proficiency. One of the primary reasons for all supervision is to ensure that the quality of therapeutic intervention with the client is of a consistently high standard in relation to the client's needs. Consequently, supervision must be acknowledged as a cornerstone of clinical practice (CPNA, 1989).

Contrary to being passive components in a system, CPNs must continually be aware of their need to forge ahead and develop the relevant skills and responses (CPNA, 1985). So what exactly is the enabling mechanism contained within the process of clinical supervision which facilitates this 'moving forward'? According to Piaget (1970), progress occurs as a result of the dual process of assimilation and accommodation. Assimilation is a process which involves the incorporation of new information into our current belief systems. Sometimes, we are unable to interlock these pieces of information into our existing belief patterns and, consequently, we must moderate extant concepts to accommodate the new data. Without this process of assimilation and accommodation the enabling circuit is incomplete and growth and development is limited. In supervision, it is the recognition of the data that does not fit which provides a trigger for assimilation and accommodation to occur. It is a constant process resulting in continuous forward movement, the final pay-off being an implementation of more effective interventions with clients (Figure 14.1).

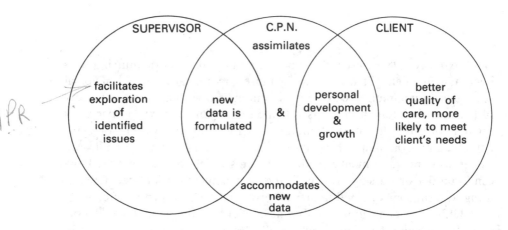

**Figure 14.1**  The 'enabling mechanism' within clinical supervision.

Fundamentally, supervision has a dualistic role within CPN work, enabling nurses to become better practitioners whilst urging exploration of areas within themselves which might be inhibiting them in practice. The supervision setting can provide a route towards this self-awareness. The facilitation of introspection by the supervisor encourages the CPN to look inside and explore his/her own feelings. This, in turn, enables an identification of both strengths and weaknesses. As weaknesses are identified and resolved, there develops a greater personal understanding. The main advantage of self-awareness is that it reduces the likelihood of over-identification with the client. If we know the reasons why we feel sad, angry or aroused, we are more able to take a step backwards and see a wider perspective of our client's problems (Burnard, 1985). Ultimately, we are now more likely to empathize accurately with our client and, consequently, be more effective in our nursing interventions. Simmons and Brooker (1986) support this philosophy by describing the aim of supervision to be: 'to facilitate the nurse in developing a different perspective on her work with clients, by encouraging greater self-awareness and building on her strengths and therapeutic and coping skills'.

Hingley and Harris (1986) propose that: 'All nurses should have access to a professional supervisor or mentor, someone within the workplace who can listen openly, challenge constructively and guide supportively'. If we are never constructively challenged about our performances, we are unlikely to recognize our weaknesses and we may well continue to function at the same level—day in, day out. Sundeen *et al.* (1985) seem to reinforce this view by suggesting that the ability to receive criticism indicates a more experienced and self-assured person, which are essential components when working within a helping profession. Supervision promotes the confidence to break away from a parochial therapeutic standpoint and facilitate a more eclectic and autonomous approach to client care. As Stoltenberg and Delworth (1987) declare: 'The purpose of supervision . . . is to foster the growth of the trainee toward a more independent functioning based on acquired skills and insight into the client and the trainee's own person'.

When supervision is introduced as a regular feature of the CPN's work it helps to serve as a preventative measure against the isolation and solitude often experienced when working in the community (Wilkin, 1988). Implementing a network of supervision within the CPN team is probably the most effective preventative measure against the self-destruction that continuous stress and lack of support inevitably leads to. By meeting the emotional needs of each individual CPN, it becomes a professional survival kit against the insidious and ever-present threat of burnout.

## THE COMPONENTS OF CLINICAL SUPERVISION

Whilst clinical supervision can be viewed as an all-embracing procedure, it does, in fact, include within it several identifiable components. The basic aims of the supervisor in each of these components is as follows:

1. Casework skills   To assist the CPN:
    a) to assess individual problems and needs;
    b) to formulate and document clinical strategies;
    c) to implement and evaluate clinical interventions;
    d) to identify alternative strategies and interventions;
    e) to improve therapeutic skills;

      f) to widen clinical knowledge base;
      g) to identify alternative and more appropriate community resources.
2.  Personal feelings  To assist the CPN:
      a) to identify feelings aroused in him by his clients or the work situation;
      b) to explore the significance and appropriateness of those feelings;
      c) to resolve negative feelings;
      d) to achieve emotional growth through self-awareness;
      e) to identify sources of personal stressors and ways of dealing with them.

Although different components of casework skills and personal feelings within the sphere of clinical supervision can be identified, there are sometimes very fine dividing lines between the two categories. Quite often, a flush of feelings will permeate the membrane which separates the two, and a behavioural issue will suddenly facilitate a very personal journey. Similarly, the self-realization of responding in a particular way in a certain situation may just as easily ignite our academic light bulbs and enlighten the appropriate therapeutic interventions in a given situation.

3.  Managerial overview
      a) to appraise regularly personal development and casework practice;
      b) to discuss and advise on caseload management;
      c) to discuss career development and further training;
      d) to discuss role responsibilities;
      e) to maintain a high morale amongst team members;
      f) to discuss personal stressors and workload pressures;
      g) to discuss and encourage research initiatives and innovative practice;
      h) to evaluate the efficacy of clinical supervision sessions.

The managerial component of clinical supervision should be governed by the CPN services' operational policy. All managerial supervisory interventions relating to the CPN's casework can be outlined in the policy and implemented accordingly. For instance, it may be agreed that each CPN will be given the opportunity to discuss his or her own career development and the appropriate further training on a yearly basis with the relevant manager, followed by a team discussion on the same subject shortly afterwards.

Whereas the two components of casework skills and personal feelings run side by side, the managerial overview is a separate component which, although of equal importance, might best be envisaged on a higher plane or at the apex of a triangle.

4.  Educative process

Throughout the whole process of clinical supervision, there is an educative process, which is an integral part of the model. Whatever the issue, emphasis during the supervisory session is on the development of increased knowledge and proficiency by the CPN. When all the various components are brought together, the whole clinical supervisory process is then enabled, and we can identify a model which can be represented as in Figure 14.2.

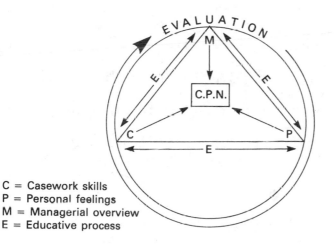

C = Casework skills
P = Personal feelings
M = Managerial overview
E = Educative process

**Figure 14.2** A model of clinical supervision for CPNs.

## THE CLINICAL SUPERVISION SESSION

If supervision is to provide a viable model with which to work, it is important to identify the boundaries which will contain both the content and process of a supervision session. Although nursing interventions are important, the emphasis of this model is on the actual supervision, so that it can be adopted as a universal approach which embraces all the CPN's clinical practice. The two categories of casework skills and personal feelings need foundation blocks on which to house the infrastructure of a supervision session. In other words, there is no point in having a supervision session if you have no idea what it is you should be supervising. These foundation blocks can be identified as Assessment, Contract, Working Alliance and Termination. To be able to conduct a supervision session effectively therefore, an outline of what these four blocks entail, together with an explanation of how they relate to the individual components, is essential.

## Assessment

Issues to be considered within the supervision session:

*Casework skills* The primary objective of an assessment is to determine if CPN intervention is appropriate. If the prospective client and the CPN fail to reach this conclusion, there is no way things should progress beyond an assessment stage. The referring agent should be contacted and informed and, if possible, more appropriate alternative helping agencies identified. Examples of issues which need to be addressed in relation to this subject are:

1.  Where did the referral come from? Did it seem to be an appropriate referral?
2.  Was your client expecting you? How did you contact your client before you saw him?
3.  Where did you see your client? Why did you decide upon that location?
4.  How did you greet your client? How did your client react to you?
5.  How did you describe your role to the client?
6.  How did your client feel about being referred to the CPN Service?
7.  How do you intend to work with this person? Do you possess the necessary skills/knowledge to be able to do so?
8.  Would other disciplines/colleagues be better able to help this person? If so, who?
9.  Did you allow your client enough time to talk about himself and his problem(s)?
10. Did you allow your client to ask questions?

*Personal feelings* No matter what happens during an assessment session with clients, it will create feelings within the nurse. Some of those feelings are readily identifiable, others are not. It is important to explore feelings in supervision to increase self-awareness and develop as a nurse practitioner. Some questions which can assist self-exploration are as follows:

1.  What were your feelings towards your client both immediately and during the assessment session?
2.  Why do you think you felt this way about your client?
3.  How did your client behave towards you during the assessment session? Why do you think this was so?

4. Do you feel able to work with this person?
5. Did you feel able to engage your client? Why do you think this was so?

Through separating certain issues into the two different categories, it is possible to see the almost invisible boundaries between them. For example, the question 'Do you feel able to work with this person?' may elicit the initial response of: 'No!'. This may be due either to realizing clinical limitations with a person (a casework skills issue) or, alternatively, taking a dislike to them (a personal feelings issue). However, if the latter reason applies, this may be due to having firstly provoked a negative response from the client at the beginning of the interview because the nurse arrived with insufficient information (a casework skills issue). On the other hand, it may have been due to being rather over-friendly at the first introduction. Obviously, the two components are often so closely related that there are large grey areas where they fuse together and become indistinguishable.

The information which needs to be collected during an assessment period will differ, depending on the therapeutic approach of the CPN. However, what is essential is the conceptualization of whatever life-problems the prospective client is experiencing, in order to determine what changes and objectives you are going to work towards.

History taking, which is included under the umbrella of assessment, is full of personal preferences, dictated to a certain degree by the way in which the individual nurse works. For example, a CPN whose roots are firmly entrenched in family therapy will, quite probably, wish to complete a genogram with the client. Similarly, if the presenting problem is a psychosexual one, the history will focus heavily on psychosexual development and other issues of sexuality. What the supervision session needs to focus on are both the content and the process of the history taking. Besides examining the information, both verbal and non-verbal, gathered during the session, the dynamics between CPN and client need to be discussed. Again, it will depend upon the reaction of the supervisee to each individual question as to which direction he sets off in. It may be that he/she responds by treading a very personal pathway or, alternatively, he/she may wish to focus on a particular skills issue. More often than not, he/she will find themselves fluctuating between the two climates throughout the supervision session. Some of the key questions which may need to be asked, albeit much less clinically than illustrated here, are:

1. Why did you do/say that?
2. Why do you think your client did/said that?
3. How else could you have phrased/done that?
4. What effect might that have had?

5. Have you considered saying/doing this . . .?
6. How do you think your client must have felt?
7. How did it make you feel?
8. How do you feel here and now?
9. Why do you think you feel this way?

Much more direct questions also need to be asked to clarify any unclear issues or to fill in any gaps.

### Contract

There are issues to be considered during the supervision session: According to Sundeen *et al.* (1985), 'The mutual establishment of a contract sets a tone for the collaborative nature of the helping relationship, in which the client participates fully in setting goals and evaluating the effectiveness of nursing interventions'.

Besides stipulating the objectives of therapy, it should also include issues such as confidentiality, time and place of sessions, expected length of therapy, when to terminate the relationship, cancelling sessions, lateness, and other ground rules or limits which either the CPN or client feel they need to impose (e.g. regular drug screening; TV must be switched off during visits; only female CPN to administer injection, etc.). Without a contract, the boundaries of the nurse–patient relationship remain woolly and prone to failure. Discussion points during supervision can relate to any aspects of the contract, not only from a clinical viewpoint (e.g. why did you insist upon random urine testing?; why are you not seeing this man together with his wife?; what will you do if your client is persistently late for sessions?) but, additionally, to the CPN's feelings about the content of the contract (e.g. how did you feel when (a) you asked for permission to request random urine samples?; (b) your client insisted that a female nurse give the injection?; (c) your client refused to let you send a letter to his doctor?).

### Working alliance

This is the actual period of work between the CPN and the client, which is determined by the contract, the CPN's approach and the client's responses. It delineates the period of time which the client and the CPN spend together, working towards the accomplishment of mutually determined goals. Supervision during the alliance stage of the nurse–patient relationship should relate to both the verbal and non-verbal contents and, of course, the process of the session. In addition to looking at communication, therefore, many other areas need to be explored.

The actual relationship between the CPN and his client will probably provide most of the material discussed within the supervision setting. If we now relate back to earlier definitions of supervision, we can perhaps highlight how it can 'promote the development of therapeutic proficiency'.

Suppose that, during a therapy session, the CPN had reached a stage where he could not identify a single therapeutic strategy to offer to his client. He had left the session feeling quite impotent and very frustrated. When he related this tale in supervision, his supervisor tentatively enquired why the CPN considered it so important to be able to offer his client a solution to her problem. The process which ensued during the remainder of the supervision session was as follows.

The CPN eventually began to realize that it was not a failing if he did not have all the answers. He began to take on board the concept that, indeed, it was quite acceptable not to know. Further exploration, facilitated by the supervisor, revealed that, as a child, the CPN's father would severely chastise him if ever he failed in his examinations at school. He had, in fact, been brainwashed into thinking that 'not knowing the answers' was synonymous with failing. During the supervision session, the realization that this was not, in fact, so had finally dawned on the CPN. Consequently, alternative responses to the client were discussed, including an open admission that he did not have any ready-made solution to the problem.

During the next therapy session, the CPN actually made this statement, to which the client replied: 'Yes. I know—I guess I was expecting you to have a magic wand, but that's totally unrealistic, isn't it?'. Not only did the client accept the CPN not having the answer, but rapport between the two of them significantly deepened after this comment—quite probably due to the CPN's openness about not having automatic solutions to problems.

What had actually happened within the supervision session was, through the 'interpersonal experience', the CPN had developed his 'therapeutic proficiency' whilst, concurrently, becoming much more self-aware. If we relate this to Piaget's theory (1970), the CPN loosened his existing assimilations (inability to solve problems = failure) and accommodated the new concept of 'it's O.K. not to know all the answers'. As soon as he was able to acknowledge that the 'failure' data did not fit, this triggered off the assimilation and accommodation.

## Termination

Issues to be covered during the supervision session: One must grant at the outset that termination is affected, or even determined, by the factors that brought the individual to therapy in the first place. When those aims have been met, it is usually time to terminate. The ultimate objective of any relationship is a satisfactory ending—the proverbial 'walk into the sunset' (parallel in its broader context with acceptance of death). A satisfactory ending depends upon both the client's past experiences and state of mind when ending is imminent and, also, the CPN's feelings regarding finishing relationships.

Quite often, the CPN harbours ambivalent feelings towards finishing the relationship, due to the impending loss that both he and his client will experience (Sundeen *et al.*, 1985). Interventions that have not been particularly helpful to the client may also complicate ending therapy ('if this fails, perhaps I am beyond help!'). Furthermore, the client is likely to regress when termination is imminent, in an attempt to prolong the inevitably painful 'goodbye'. Exploration of what termination may entail within specific, CPN–client relationships can be effected during supervision and any projected or actual difficulties can be discussed and often resolved.

SUPERVISORY SKILLS

## Communication skills

Communication is the key to effective supervision. Besides being attentive and actively listening to what is said during a supervision session, there are a number of other important, core concepts. The supervisor must be able to comment openly, objectively and constructively if he is to gain the respect of the supervisee. Similarly, suggestions as opposed to dogmatic pieces of advice should be offered as tentative options. Likewise, positive feedback should be given when appropriate. Questions need to be asked when necessary and situations clarified and/or interpreted when the need arises.

It is, of course, very important that feelings are verbalized and an effective supervisor is able to facilitate the expression of feelings and support the supervisee if need be. Ultimately, examination of feelings and responses leads to a greater self-understanding and are a catalyst for personal growth.

## Supportive skills

Sometimes, there are moments when the supervisor's biggest asset is her availability during the supervision session. The CPN is not looking for any direction, nor any earth-shattering interventions. Purely and simply, he is in need of support. To be able to provide that support, the primary skills which the supervisor needs are identification, spontaneity and genuineness. It is an acquired skill to be able to identify when the giving of support is appropriate. When it is, it must be a spontaneous gesture with 'no strings attached'—a genuine response which radiates the message: 'I understand and I am with you'. Supportive responses are an essential ingredient in the supervisor's repertory, in that they are able to soak up emotions from within the CPN which, if unventilated, could eventually fester and prove detrimental to his mental health. In this sense, it can be seen as a means of professional survival for the CPN.

## General skills

Community psychiatric nursing is a very specialized area of nursing which, if it is to be performed effectively, requires a specific knowledge base and certain core skills. Consequently, with the exception of certain clinical specialties, only people who possess these qualifications are in a position to provide clinical supervision for CPNs. This, in turn, highlights the importance of the ENB approved course in 'Nursing Care of Mentally Ill People in the Community' which, although not a mandatory course, is the only recognized training course provided for CPNs. Even though experienced CPNs without this qualification are able to supervise each other, it would seem to make more sense if all CPNs were to undergo the same comprehensive foundation course, which would provide them with a similar platform from which to develop themselves.

## Specialist skills

If a CPN has decided to specialize in either a particular field and/or a specific therapeutic approach, then it makes sense to seek supervision from someone who is similarly orientated (Pollock, 1988). This may mean receiving supervision from outside the team, or even from another discipline. Not only is this perfectly acceptable practice, it must be actively encouraged to ensure that the most effective supervision is available to each individual CPN. It is strongly recommended, however, that you include the provision of outside supervision as a viable option in your operational policy.

### OTHER REQUIREMENTS IN CLINICAL SUPERVISION

## Mandate

If supervision is to formulate the basis for a CPN's actions, then it should be included in the team's Operational Policy. Consequently, this provides a mandate, or 'permission to act', from management, officially recognizing supervision as an integral part of the CPN's working week. Without it, supervision could be interpreted as an optional exercise, which would diminish the credibility and, of course, the efficacy of such a model.

## Local resources

If all people referred to CPN services are to be offered the best available method of resolving their own, unique problems, the effective supervisor must be aware of all the available local resources. It is one thing being able to identify needs that cannot be met by the designated CPN, it is equally as important to be aware of all the other options and resources which the client may need to be made aware of.

## Local policy and philosophy of the service

An understanding of the service's philosophy is absolutely essential as, without such knowledge, there can be no theoretical foundation to underpin decisions. Within a supervisory setting, such a lack of knowledge would devalue all the interventions of the supervisor.

## Supervisory milieu

Far from being an ad hoc exercise, supervision should be officially slotted into a CPN's modus operandi. If it is to form the basis of clinical practice, it must be a permanent feature of each working week. It can be helpful to draw up a contract which contains the ground rules for every session. Within these regulations should be the agreed location, time and duration of sessions. Other issues which need to be considered within such a contract are confidentiality, relating particularly to the revelation of personal feelings (the confidentiality of clinical material goes without saying), how time is to be allocated during each session and, perhaps, whether the content and/or process of the sessions is to be officially documented afterwards. There are a number of advantages for documenting the clinical content of supervision sessions. Besides contributing more information in the nursing notes, it can also be related to as a learning experience at a later date. Furthermore, it would be foolish to spend time discussing a particular case and eventually forget what had been said, particularly if the case is still open.

It is important, therefore, not merely to pay lip-service to the concept of supervision but to ensure that, wherever possible, we turn our words into the kind of actions that will, ultimately, be of benefit to our clients.

Finally, a few words about the environment in which the supervision sessions take place. There needs to be a room which is always available and where there is likely to be neither noise nor any interruptions or disturbances (preferably without a telephone). The room should be booked in advance if need be to ensure the sessions can start on time and any teaching aids which have been identified as essential to the session provided. Obviously, there needs to be adequate, comfortable seating for all the people present.

The room itself needs to be aesthetically decorated and of a comfortable temperature in order to promote a pleasant feeling amongst its occupants. A poky, shabby and sparsely furnished room that feels like an oven is certainly not conducive to a working environment.

## HOW CAN SUPERVISION BE PROVIDED?

There are several ways in which supervision sessions can be organized within a CPN service:

1. Peer supervision, either on a one-to-one basis or within a small group setting; the obvious advantage is that the universal identification provided by peer supervision provides a sound platform from which to launch supervision sessions. The team leader or manager's role in peer supervision is purely a monitoring exercise. They would not be included in the actual supervision session.
2. Team supervision, which involves focusing on the team objectives as opposed to individual work. Usually facilitated by one identified supervisor.
3. Shadow supervision  One nurse, possibly a student or a newly appointed CPN undertaking an induction programme, is attached as a shadow to an experienced CPN to learn by observation.
4. Managerial or tutorial supervision  The team leader supervises an individual student of CPN formally and privately.
5. Pair supervision, which involves two CPNs being supervised by their team leader or manager.

Supervision can also be carried out in vivo, during the actual nurse/ client meeting, after which it is discussed between the two supervision partners.

Whilst the above examples are founded on the basis of a conversation between supervision partners, experiential learning techniques can also be implemented by employing such methods as role playing, structured exercises and games.

## Choosing Your Supervision Partner(s)

The important factors for selecting a supervision partner seem to be mutual trust, respect for each other and feeling comfortable in each other's presence. It is immensely gratifying to know that there is a colleague who is not only willing to sit and listen to you but who will 'climb in there with you'. In a study by Firth *et al.* (1986) concerning interpersonal support between nurses, they concluded that supervisors who emanated empathy and respect contributed significantly to reduced 'emotional exhaustion' amongst those being supervised. Additionally, it is equally important that a supervisor possesses the skills and knowledge required to enable him to supervise effectively. If the supervisee does not recognize any of the above qualities in his partner, the supervision will be ineffectual.

It may be argued (and frequently is!) that supervision has been practised within community psychiatric nursing for many years: 'We have supervision every day' is one commonly heard cry; 'We always discuss difficult cases when we get back to the office'. It is a natural and understandable reaction to want to 'unload' immediately after a particularly intense session with a client. And who better to dump your excess baggage with than your colleagues, who know all about such stressful and frustrating sessions and who appreciate the importance of confidentiality in nursing? This basic instinct to share thoughts and feelings with our peers is a built-in safety valve, which prevents problems and intense emotions from bubbling away inside us for long periods.

However, although these extemporary encounters employ some of the principles behind supervision, such spontaneous, unstructured interactions can never be classed as clinical supervision. Unless the specified structure explained throughout this chapter is implemented, the process is not complete and the enabling function is not possible.

## SUMMARY

Whilst advocating clinical supervision as being the very lifeblood of CPN work, it is essential that we view it in a facilitative context as opposed to being somewhat of an imposition. Indeed, supervision should be an unshackling process—an opening of previously locked doors. Far from being a corrective experience, which conjures up images of brandished canes and books stuffed down trousers, it should be seen as an exploratory relationship in an environment which aids development and promotes change. Supervision should not be an invasion of inner privacy but a much more tentative and empathic exercise. Supervision should be, essentially, non-threatening enough to ensure participation, yet challenging and stimulating enough to encourage exploration. On the one hand, we owe it to our clients in the community to provide the best possible service to them. It is scrutinizing and evaluating our actions. Furthermore, it is tremendously conceited to think that we can effectively evaluate our own interventions in a totally objective manner. On the other hand, if we never considered the emotions created within us by client contact, we would learn very little about what it is that makes us as individuals tick. Nor would we be able to confront our own neuroses and develop healthier and more helpful ways of responding to our clients.

Finally, we would not be looking after ourselves as we should if we allowed ourselves to be frequently consumed by the stresses that we encounter whilst carrying out our job. Sharing these stressful feelings in supervision can release personal tension whilst, concurrently, identifying ways of counteracting stressful situations.

It is insufficient that clinical supervision is merely introduced as a baseline for all CPN practice. This particular CPN model, as with all models, needs to be implemented and continuously evaluated if it is to become an effective and credible approach to community care. Additionally, a viable model of clinical supervision which can be employed by all CPNs should be incorporated into all current and future approved courses for CPNs and a policy statement published and distributed to all practising CPNs and their managers by the Community Psychiatric Nurses Association.

## REFERENCES

Burnard, P. (1985) *Learning Human Skills: A Guide for Nurses*, Heinemann, London.

Community Psychiatric Nurses Association (1985) *The Clinical Nursing Responsibilities of the C.P.N.*, C.P.N.A. Publications.

Community Psychiatric Nurses Association (1989) *Clinical Practice Issues for C.P.N.s*, C.P.N.A. Publications.

Firth, H., McIntee, J., McKeown, P. and Britton, P. (1986) Interpersonal support amongst nurses at work, *Journal of Advanced Nursing*, **11**, 273–282.

Hingley, P. and Harris, P. (1986) Lowering the tension, *Nursing Times*, 6 August, 52–53.

Piaget, J. (1970) *Structuralism*, Basic Books, New York.

Pollock, L. (1988) The future work of community psychiatric nursing, *Community Psychiatric Nursing Journal*, **8**(5), 5–13.

Simmons, S. and Brooker, C. (1986) *Community Psychiatric Nursing; A Social Perspective*, Heinemann, London.

Skidmore, D. and Friend, W. (1984) Muddling through, *Nursing Times, Community Outlook*, 9 May, 179–181.

Stoltenberg, C. D. and Delworth, U. (1987) *Supervising Counselors and Therapists; A Developmental Approach*, Jossey-Bass, San Francisco.

Sundeen, S. J., Stuart, G. W., Rankin, E. D. and Cohen, S. A. (1985) *Nurse–Client Interaction*, Mosby, St Louis.

Wilkin, P. (1988) Someone to watch over me, *Nursing Times*, 17 August, **84**(33), 33–34.

# PART THREE

# Developmental Perspectives

## INTRODUCTION

The concluding part of this book consists of two chapters which explore ideas which relate to the area of clinical supervision and mentorship and yet cannot be fixed within any one specialty of nursing, and a final chapter which proposes a framework for clinical supervision and mentorship.

Steve Wright presents a chapter in which he recommends the role of 'consultant nurse' as a provider of clinical excellence and supervision to those who are practising at an advanced level. This model allows the notion of clinical supervision to extend beyond the realms of student teaching and preceptorship for the newly qualified.

Jean Faugier follows with a chapter which is an account of exchanges between nurses and their supervisors. The examples she gives are from situations which are to be found by many nurses in their day-to-day practice and show the way in which nurses' own experiences, feelings and values are drawn into work situations and relationships with users and patients.

Finally we present a model for 'supervision for life'. Taking a variety of ideas expressed in various parts of this book we have sought to weld them into a grand design of possibilities. This is not an end point but merely a beginning whereby we hope that others will challenge, modify and if necessary reject the ideas we put forward. That is the process of development and change from which we shall all grow.

# CHAPTER FIFTEEN

# Modelling excellence: the role of the consultant nurse

*Steve Wright*

## INTRODUCTION—WHO IS THE CONSULTANT?

The use of the term 'consultant' is widespread in many occupations. It refers usually to a person who has acquired specialist knowledge and skills, and to whom others refer for advice. Within the health sphere however, the word until recently has been almost exclusively the province of doctors. Some might argue that when nurses attach this title to their role, it is an attempt to take on board some of the aura of the power and status of medicine. Hostility from both nurses and doctors might be expected as a result.

On the other hand, there appears to be no reason for a word to be monopolized by one discipline. In recent years many nurses have offered their expertise, usually working privately as individuals or part of larger companies and associations, as consultants in a wide range of issues of health care. From setting up conferences to advising on nursing practice in a nursing home, from planning and conducting staff development courses to advising industry on nursing issues—the range of activities in which nurses have become involved as consultants is extensive. Many have specifically used the term 'consultant nurse', 'nurse consultant' or 'consultants in nursing' to describe what they do. The plethora of roles in which nurses 'consult' has led to difficulties over definitions.

Within the National Health Service, relatively few roles appear to have been created with the specific 'consultant' title. However, perhaps because of inter-professional sensitivities over the word, many nurses act in a consultancy capacity while not necessarily including the word in their job title. Nurse managers, teachers, clinical specialists, sisters and charge nurses, for example, quite commonly have a consultation role in giving advice on nursing practice to others. It will be argued in this chapter that the traditional model of the consultant has limitations when considering the desired influence over supervision, learning and innovation in the clinical setting. To enhance control over these elements, the consultant role has to be developed to incorporate key aspects of clinical practice, i.e. involvement in and direct accountability for 'hands-on' nursing.

Caplan (1970) has identified four basic types of consultation:

1. Nurse-centred, e.g. a primary nurse seeks advice from a consultant nurse on the management of a specific patient's problem. (There is advice to the nurse but no direct involvement with the patient.)
2. Patient-centred, e.g. several nurses ask the consultant to work with them to manage the care of a particular patient. (The advice to nurses encompasses working with the patient.)
3. Programme-centred, e.g. planning staff development courses.
4. Administration-centred, e.g. giving advice to management on nursing policy and practice.

In practice, circumstances are rarely so linear and it may be that more than one of these overlaps at any one time.

Menard (1987) sees the consultant as (trained) teacher and expert in a particular specialty. Boehm (1956), however, adds that the consultant remains relatively distant from the problem—someone whose advice may be sought, but with a 'take it or leave it' quality on the part of the recipient. Pearson (1983) and Wright (1986) have laid greater emphasis on the consultant nurse being directly involved in practice, working as a skilled change agent and educator. They agree with Benner (1984) that the consultant nurse needs to have considerable post-graduate experience and education—at least to masters degree level. This nurse has become not only an expert in nursing practice but has learned to work within the organization and use 'a variety of creative ways of getting around the bureaucracy' to meet the needs of nurse, patients and families. The roles are often 'broader and more complex' (Benner, 1984) than can be defined by the job description, as the expert nurse works both formally and informally to affect practice, and is involved in both monitoring and evaluating the outcome.

Johnson et al. (1989) described the creation of a consultant nurse's role. The post-holder was specifically required to be a registered nurse tutor and master (in nursing) graduate as well as having other relevant qualifications and experience. The role was envisaged as a change agent who would continue the development of nursing and nurses. Some of the general aims of the post were noted as:

    to retain a senior nurse with a high level of clinical, educational, research and management expertise at clinical level;

to demonstrate and encourage excellence in nursing;

to support the conduct of nursing research at clinical level and application of findings;

to act as a resource person to clinical nurses and senior management as an expert in nursing practice for the elderly patient. (Johnson *et al.*, 1989)

These main aims fall broadly within the range of what might be deemed as the consultant nurse's role where it is desirable to have a direct effect on practice. The well educated expert nurse, working within the organization as teacher, practitioner and change agent, appears to be in a suitable position to act as a consultant in clinical nursing and for clinical nurses.

## THE QUALITIES OF THE NURSE AS CONSULTANT

While considerable emphasis has been placed on the appropriate knowledge and expertise of the consultant nurse, the qualities which that person possesses also need to be examined. From Pearson (1983 and 1985), Wright (1986 and 1989), Ottoway (1980) and Roy and Martinez (1983) a number of key features can be further identified:

- possessor of mature clinical or professional judgement
- a highly developed sense of accountability
- articulate, both verbally and in writing
- sensitivity and objectivity with decision-making skills
- high levels of inter-personal and communication skills
- physical and psychological stamina
- analytical thinking abilities
- ability to use initiative
- awareness of self, abilities, limitations, etc.
- high level of commitment to nurses and nursing

When these features are combined with the education and experience and expert practitioner qualities, it might be wondered if sufficient numbers of individuals exist to meet these demanding requirements. Benner (1984) argues that many nurses have the capacity to operate at this level.

However, large parts of the present educational and organizational structures of nursing appear to militate against the development of such nurses (RCN, 1986). Part of the response, in British nursing, has been to undertake wholesale changes in the nursing education system in order to produce more questioning and creative practitioners (UKCC, 1986). A recent King's fund project (Scutari, 1989) aims to support units which foster learning in nursing and produce new roles for clinical leaders. Meanwhile, there are signs that increasing numbers of degree course places for nurses and an expansion of nursing departments in Polytechnics and Universities are under way.

To support the consultant nurses in their work, it is clear that they too have requirements (Roy and Martinez, 1983; Johnson *et al.*, 1989), specifically for peer group and managerial support, opportunities for continued education, clarity of their expectations and their position in the organization and adequate secretarial facilities. Such support is not, of course, unique to consultant nurses, but it is a pre-requisite to enable the consultant nurse to be free to practise in situations which demand a high degree of flexibility and spontaneity. Kafka (1916) notes that 'sometimes it is safer to be in chains than to be free'. The freedom of wider professional horizons which the consultant nurse enjoys must be adequately defined and resourced in a variety of ways if the consultant nurse role is not to lapse into that of ineffectual bureaucrat or become burned out.

## THE CONSULTANT AS PRACTITIONER

A key role for the consultant in nursing is to bring expertise to the day-to-day practice world of nurses. However, it is not sufficient merely to be present with nurses in the workplace, offer advice, and then retreat from the work setting. In this sense, the consultant in being clinically involved is a move away from the model of the consultant as an aloof and uncommitted figure. Encouraging learning, motivating nurses, sharing expertise and acting as a role model for others to follow can only take place in a setting which positively encourages these behaviours. Being directly involved in the workplace enables the consultant to be instrumental in producing the climate for learning, innovation and the achievement of high quality care. If the consultant nurse remains aloof from practice, there are considerable risks to the achievement of his or her goals. Clearly, to function as a role model for excellence (defined in the dictionary as 'having merit or worth' or 'surpassing others in good quality') is difficult if the consultant is not present with nurses for more than brief periods of advice. Nursing, as a practice discipline, needs experts who cannot only describe theory or help with the solving of problems, but who can also demonstrate a desired approach in practice. Benner and Wrubel (1989) have described 'presencing'—the ability of the nurse to 'be with' the patient, to sympathize, empathize and to promote healing and learning through therapeutic nursing. Campbell (1984) uses the term 'companionship' to describe the role of the nurse in helping the patient to heal, to learn or to change his or her lifestyle.

It seems that there are similarities between the relationship which needs to exist between consultant and nurse, and that between nurse and patient. Being a 'presence' with the nurse or group or nurses, acting as companion or guide through the processes of learning, helping and changing, underpin the ability of the consultant to act as a role model. Rogers (1983), Hurst (1985) and the English National Board (1987), for example, seem to suggest that a similar role for the educator emerges where it is desirable that there is a direct effect upon practice.

The ability to demonstrate excellence in practice, and the opportunity to bring to the clinical setting the expertise that can only be acquired over many years of learning, are fundamental to the value and role of the consultant nurse. To be divorced from practice would expose the consultant to the risk of being seen as an 'ivory tower' nurse reinforcing, not bridging, the gap between the theory and practice of nursing. Where the consultant nurse has a role which requires immediate effect upon practice, and those nurses involved in it, it is essential that they remain a clinician. This might take the form of working with nurses and patients over quite long periods of time and perhaps taking full responsibility for the care of some patients as a primary or associate nurse.

Whatever the method chosen, having some degree of accountability for patient care puts the consultant nurse in the best position to influence colleagues and retain clinical credibility.

## THE CONSULTANT NURSE AND THE BOUNDARIES OF NURSING

As an active participant in the clinical field, the consultant nurse has other attributes which offer a model of excellence to others. This nurse has a very clear 'image' in his or her head (Reilly, 1975) of what nursing is. This defining of their nursing model enables them to use a systematic problem-solving approach to their work, to practise on the basis of sound knowledge and to transform relationships with patients and colleagues.

The consultant nurse has both the knowledge and skill to promote care which is personalized and patient-centred, not ritualized or institutionalized. A nurse of this calibre is in the vanguard of what Salvage (1990) has called the 'new nursing'. The key to this is considered to be its clinical base where 'the bureaucratic occupational model must be replaced by a professional one, with the practitioner as its linchpin, prepared to fulfil her responsible, skilled and demanding role through an improved educational programme. This "new animal" should have greater autonomy at the centre of a new division of labour' (Salvage, 1990).

Consultants in nursing, it seems, are some of that breed of 'new animal' who have taken on board a renewed vision of what nursing is. They expand the concept of the 'unique function' (Henderson, 1966) of the nurse into the territory where nursing is recognized as a healing, therapeutic act in its own right (Pearson *et al.*, 1988).

The concept of the expanding role of the nurse is different from that of extension. Each has different sets of values underpinning it. The expanded role, for example, rejects the notion that some aspects of care are 'menial' or 'basic' (which can then be devoted to the untrained or partially trained support worker). There is a recognition that such acts are highly intricate, complex and skilful and have an intrinsic therapeutic component. Extension of the nurse's role usually means accepting certain tasks delegated by medicine, usually of a technical nature. Often such tasks have been developed because of inadequate medical resources (e.g. the nurse being asked to give intravenous drugs because the doctor is busy elsewhere). At other times it may be because nurses themselves have been lured by what Oakley (1984) has described as the 'narcissistic mirror offered by medicine'. In this instance nurses have come to value aspects of health care associated with the status and scientific 'high-tech' cure aspects of medicine.

In so doing, there is a risk that they may ignore the importance of the expressive side of nursing—the 'high touch' approach which embodies the nurse's caring and therapeutic function and which enables them to fulfil the role which patients expect of them, that of humanizing the health care system. Holder (1989) has summarized some of these issues:

**The expanding role**

- nursing practices which develop and build on the fundamental role to promote healing;
- skills which promote patient/client independence and health education;
- caring skills, which give nurture and succour, counselling and advocacy;
- analytical skills based on sound knowledge;
- restorative skills, which may include some technical and medical treatments aimed at rehabilitation;

**The extended role**

- practices, delegated medical or other professionals, not previously embedded in the nurse's fundamental role;
- usually technical in nature;
- may be acquired over time or may require specific training.

It is part of the role of consultant nurse to help define those areas of nursing where expansion or extension is taking place, and to help colleagues do likewise. Where extension occurs, is it to make care more holistic or to satisfy some need in the nurse for dubious status or to resolve the inadequate resources of other disciplines? There is an inherent tension between what Benner (1984) has described as the 'expressive' role of the nurse (the being with, 'presencing' skills which help heal the patient) and the instrumental skills (the carrying out of technical procedures forming part of the patient's treatment and care). Arguments have tended to polarize around the notions of expansion and extension, with 'fors' and 'againsts' gathering in both camps. Perhaps the challenge for nurses, and specifically of those in clinical leaderships roles such as the consultant nurse, is to test out these boundaries, and to illuminate where merger and demarcation are appropriate. Thus they will help both themselves, other colleagues and their patients towards a clearer definition of their role. In this way, the consultant nurse can contribute to the generation of models and theories in nursing out of practice and help colleagues build models of care which best suit them and the patients.

## CREATING THE LEARNING CLIMATE

Pearson (1983) has described the role of the clinical nurse consultant who not only has responsibilities for nursing practice but who leads the teaching and supervision of the nursing staff. He or she may lead the 'Clinical Nursing Unit' (Pearson, 1983) or the 'Nursing Development Unit' (Salvage, 1989; Johnson *et al.*, 1991). Functioning specifically as a teacher, courses, conferences, workshops, etc., are planned which meet staff needs. There may also be involvement in helping them with open learning programmes (Robinson, 1989), with 'learning contracts' (Keyser, 1986) or with careers and personal counselling—using in fact, a whole range of educational strategies.

Apart from the practicalities of organizing a variety of teaching and development programmes, the consultant nurse can be in a significant position to influence the whole climate in which learning and innovation take place. Schweer (1972) argues that 'if we truly seek to keep creativity alive, we must continue to nourish the conditions in which creativity flourishes'. As a clinical leader, role model and expert, the consultant nurse can be in an ideal position to set the style and tone of a setting. Orton (1980), for example, defined the learning climate and its effects upon students, and noted the key role of the ward sister/charge nurse in determining that climate. Learners feeling supported, free to enquire and use initiative, and apply theory to practice are some of the hallmarks of the learning climate. Martin (1984) identified the need for leadership and expertise at clinical level to make practice innovative and supportive of learning. The 'clinical laboratory' (Infante, 1985) has to be created to allow staff at all levels to continue their learning and to experiment in nursing, yet within safe limits for both nurses and patients.

The consultant nurse, as a clinical leader can provide the supervision which supports freedom to practise, yet, by using expertise, protects both nurse and patient. The concept of the clinical laboratory does not offer a licence for anarchy, rather it suggests an environment where learning and creativity flourish under careful guidance and supervision.

Benner (1984) likens this setting to a school for pilots. It would be rather dangerous to let the novice pilot have complete freedom at the controls of the aircraft. Working as co-pilot to the expert who encourages and supervises learning is a relatively safe way to develop expertise without putting pilot and passengers (in this case nurse and patients) at risk. A significant proportion of the acquisition of skills in nursing is not through the classroom, but by working with expert role models who demonstrate excellence in practice.

Wong's (1979) study illustrates the behaviours for those teachers and supervisors which nurses find helpful to learning, and which seem to be relevant to the role of the consultant nurse in producing a climate for learning:

**Helpful qualities**
- demonstrating willingness to answer questions and offer explanations;
- being interested in students and respectful to them;
- giving encouragement and praise;
- informing of progress;
- having an appropriate sense of humour;
- having a pleasant voice;
- being available when needed;
- giving appropriate supervision;
- displaying confidence in themselves and students.

**Qualities which hinder learning**
- posing a threat;
- being sarcastic;
- acting in a superior manner;
- belittling students;
- correcting students in the presence of others;
- supervising too closely;
- emphasizing mistakes and weaknesses. (Wong, 1979)

In the light of these points and discussion earlier in this chapter, it is clear that the consultant nurse must have a variety of positive attributes which encourage others to learn and to make use of their expertise, and to set the standard for the whole climate in which learning can take place.

When such a climate is not achieved (and all nurses in leadership positions, not just consultants have a part to play in nourishing that climate), then the ramifications go beyond the effects upon staff learning. The 'Magnet' study in the USA (McLure *et al.*, 1983) mirrors that of the Price Waterhouse (1988) report. A climate which is hostile to learning, which does not support innovative, patient-centred practice, and where managers and other leaders do not actively support staff, ultimately fails both nurses and patients. Care tends to decline to an institutional mould, and staff demonstrate their dissatisfaction with poor motivation and high sickness, absenteeism and leaving rates. Potential recruits can easily sense such a negative climate, and will seek work elsewhere, those who already work there will tend not to stay long.

Salvage (1990) has suggested that nursing has a great need of 'clinical leaders' to produce climates for creativity on a mass scale in all areas of nursing. Both nurses and nursing, and ultimately patients, would benefit by exposure to more nurses who can demonstrate expertise and excellence in their fields. However, many nurses still seem to be denied such opportunities. Many are still expected to learn through the mock-apprenticeship system of attachment to 'preceptors', whose roles and qualities may not have been clearly defined and who have not necessarily moved beyond competent to expert practitioner.

Benner (1984) argues that such experts are critical to the development of nursing practice, and consultant nurses are one avenue to enable nurses to meet up with such expertise. How far the recently applied clinical grading structures will encourage nurses to remain 'at the bedside' remains uncertain. Meanwhile, the drain of expert nurses into management or educational roles appears to continue. As Jarvis and Gibson (1985) point out, 'it does need to be recognised from the outset that those managers and teachers who no longer actually practise in the clinical situation are non-effective in this respect, within the occupation'.

There appears to be a role for application and extension of the principles of consultancy in nursing. A further avenue can be provided which permits those who have developed high levels of expertise to have a direct impact on nursing practice. The use of the consultant nurse as a role model for excellence can facilitate practice which is creative and patient-centred. Being a consultant to others is an intrinsic part of many nursing roles. Creating posts for experts with this as their specific remit has the potential to benefit both nurses and patients.

## REFERENCES

Benner, P. (1984) *From Novice to Expert*, Addison Wesley, New York.
Benner, P. and Wrubel, J. (1989) *The Primacy of Caring: Stress and Coping in Death and Illness*, Addison Wesley, Menlo Park, California.

Boehm, W. (1956) The professional relationship between consultant and consultee, *American Journal of Orthopsychiatry*, **26**, 241–248.

Campbell, A. V. (1984) *Moderated Love*, SPCK, London.

Caplan, G. (1970) *The Theory and Practice of Mental Health Consultation*, Basic Books, New York.

E.N.B. (1987) *Managing Change in Nursing Education*, English National Board for Nursing, Midwifery and Health Visitors, London.

Henderson, V. (1966) *The Nature of Nursing*, Macmillan, New York.

Holder, S. (1989) Expanding role, *Nursing Standard*, **38**(3), 52.

Hurst, K. (1985) Traditional versus progressive nurse education: a review of the literature, *Nurse Education Today*, **5**, 103–8.

Infante, M. S. (1985) *The Clinical Laboratory in Nursing Education*, Wiley, Chichester.

Jarvis, P. and Gibson, S. (1985) *The Teacher–Practitioner in Nursing, Midwifery and Health Visiting*, Croom Helm, Beckenham.

Johnson, M. L., Purdy, E. and Wright, S. G. (1991) The nurse as consultant, *Nursing Standard*, **5**(20), 31–6.

Kafka, F. (1916) *Metamorphosis*, reprinted (1974) in Penguin, Harmondsworth.

Keyser, D. M. (1986) Using learning contracts to support change in nursing organisations, *Nurse Education Today*, **6**, 103–108.

Martin, J. P. (1984) *Hospitals in Trouble*, Blackwell, London.

McLure, M. L., Poulin, M. A., Sovie, M. D. and Wandelt, M. A. (1983) *Magnet Hospitals – Attraction and Retention of Professional Nurses*, American Academy of Nursing, Kansas City.

Menard, S. N. (1987) *The Clinical Nurse Specialist – Perspectives on Practice*, Wiley, Chichester.

Oakley, A. (1984) The importance of being a nurse, *Nursing Times*, **80**(50), 24–27.

Orton, H. (1980) *The Ward Learning Climate*, RCN, London.

Ottoway, R. N. (1980) *Defining the Change Agent*, Unpublished Research Paper, University of Manchester Institute of Technology, Department of Managerial Sciences.

Pearson, A. (1983) *The Clinical Nursing Unit*, Heinemann, London.

Pearson, A. (1985) The effects of introducing new norms in a nursing unit; an analysis of the process of change, Unpublished Ph.D. Thesis, Goldsmiths College, University of London.

Pearson, A., Durand, I. and Punton, S. (1988) *Therapeutic nursing: an evaluation of an experimental nursing unit in the British National Health Service*, Burford and Oxford Nursing Development Unit, Oxford.

Price Waterhouse (1988) *Nurse Retention and Recruitment*, Price Waterhouse, London.

Reilly, D. (1975) Why a conceptual framework? *Nursing Outlook*, **23**(9), 14–22.

Robinson, K. (Ed.) (1989) *Open and Distance Learning for Nurses*, Longman, Harlow.

Rogers, C. (1983) *Freedom to Learn for the 80's*, Merrill, New York.

Roy, C. and Martinez, C. (1983) A conceptual framework for C.N.S. practice, in

*The Clinical Nurse Specialist in Theory and Practice* (A. B. Hamric and J. Spross, Eds), Grune and Stratton, Orlando, Florida.

Royal College of Nurses (1986) *The Education of Nurses: a new dispensation*, Royal College of Nursing, London.

Salvage, J. (1989) Nursing Development Units, *Nursing Standard*, **3**(22), 25.

Salvage, J. (1990) The theory and practice of the 'new nursing', *Nursing Times*, **86**(4), 42–45.

Schweer, J. E. (1972) *Creative Teaching in Clinical Nursing*, Mosby, St Louis.

United Kingdom Central Council for Nursing, Midwifery and Health Visiting (1986) *Project 2000*, UKCCN, London.

Wong, S. (1979) Nurse teacher behaviours in the clinical field: Apparent effects on nursing students' learning, *Journal of Advanced Nursing*, **3**, 369–378.

Wright, S. G. (1986) *Building and Using a Model of Nursing*, Arnold, London.

Wright, S. G. (1989) *Changing Nursing Practice*, Arnold, London.

# CHAPTER SIXTEEN

# Casework conversations

*Jean Faugier*

In this chapter, the aim is to examine the process of supervision in nursing by taking examples from real supervision sessions where the focus has been upon facilitating nurses to deal with their work. Attempts are made to analyse the interactions between supervisor and supervisee. For this reason, the focus of the cases presented here is the supervisory relationship, and not an attempt to show exemplary practice, although there are hopefully no examples of poor practice either.

## CASEWORK CONVERSATION ONE

### Background

Sheila is a staff nurse working with the elderly on what is rapidly changing from an acute medical ward to an elderly care unit. Many of the nurses with whom Sheila works have some problems with this, seeing care of the elderly as simply another word for geriatrics and a subsequent loss of status. Sheila does not share this view; she has always enjoyed nursing the elderly and has a very positive view of the old person as her mother and father are in their seventies and are both fit, well and active. Always seeking to improve her knowledge and skills, Sheila has enrolled for a 'Care of the Elderly' course which is run by her health authority. One of the conditions of the course is that students must bring casework to supervision each week. Sheila has been working with an elderly man called Ted recently and, untypically for her, she has found herself becoming increasingly irritated with him. Feeling a little confused about this patient, she decides to discuss the case in supervision.

## Supervision session one

**Sheila**:   Ted was admitted a couple of weeks ago; he is only 64 which is relatively young for our ward! Apparently, he had been having attacks of breathlessness and chest pains for a week before he was admitted. The original diagnosis was a possible myocardial infarction, but all the tests have proved nothing. The consultant has ordered some additional investigations; he isn't convinced that there is nothing wrong with Ted. Obviously, it is difficult to say, but he is such a moaner. He never seems to do a thing to help himself or anyone else, simply wants to lie in bed doing nothing all day. He won't even make an effort to move when we change him or make his bed. And trying to keep him out of bed, sitting in a chair, is a major battle of wills. What's even worse is that he is not even grateful for everything people do for him, the nurses, his family, the other patients.

**Supervisor**:   He certainly sounds as if he is getting on your nerves; I wonder what you feel he should be grateful for?

**Sheila**:   Well, he is so much younger than all our other patients and so far we have not been able to find anything wrong with him, which is more than I can say for some of the others. Quite a lot of them have terminal conditions which are quite distressing.

**Supervisor**:   So you want him to be grateful for being 64, in hospital, with us not being able to tell him why he feels bad. Perhaps you think that he in fact has no right to feel like that, especially as there has been no investigative findings showing why he should do so.

**Sheila**:   I can't see how he should feel that bad; his family come in all the time, he gets a lot of attention.

**Supervisor**:   Apart from his physical investigations and care, do you spend any time talking to him?

**Sheila**:   To be honest, I spend more of my time with two of the very elderly patients who I know are dying and need a great deal of physical attention. One of them is so frail now, all we can do is to prevent her from developing pressure sores. And frankly, I find Ted grumpy and ill mannered, and I think why should I waste my time? I have tried to talk to him about what he should be doing to keep active but he just tells me to go away. I have always thought I had a 'way' with old people, but I don't seem to get anywhere with him.

**Supervisor**:   You seem to have very strong views about Ted keeping active and doing things.

**Sheila**: My parents are both in their seventies and do everything for themselves. They go rambling on the moors in Yorkshire, and do a lot of gardening. My father goes swimming three times a week. They are totally independent and fit and healthy. My mother does more housework than me!

**Supervisor**: That's wonderful, it's great when we can avoid the nasty bits of getting old. Illness, dependence, depression, loneliness, feeling useless, feeling frightened of dying or of having to rely on someone. I wonder if you have ever thought that some of these feelings may be bothering Ted. You seem to have concentrated on getting him to do things, rather than looking at how he really feels. I suppose people like Ted upset us because they don't play the game as well as your parents. Old age is fine, but only if we don't really have to face it.

**Sheila**: I suppose I do worry about what would happen if my parents couldn't cope as well as they do. I am an only child, you see, and I would probably have to give up my job to look after them.

**Supervisor**: I wonder how that might make you feel. Are you at all worried by that possibility? You do seem to have a big investment in them keeping going.

**Sheila**: Well, I would simply have to look after them, there isn't anyone else. Although I would really hate moving back home. I suppose I would feel resentful; yes, quite resentful. But if they were really ill, if they were dying, you have to look after your parents, don't you? I mean, it's your duty.

**Supervisor**: So you have a duty as a daughter and a duty as a nurse and they are both easier to fulfil if you feel people really need you, if for example they are actually dying. If things are not, or don't seem to be, that serious, then you might feel resentful?

**Sheila**: Well, there is often so little time on the ward, we can be so busy and Ted is so demanding. I must admit that I have been a bit abrupt with him sometimes. I suppose I feel that the other patients have greater needs; after all, we are not sure why he is there. Yet the consultant has ordered tests which will mean he is staying at least another ten days.

**Supervisor**: Well, as you have got that time, I wonder if you might approach him differently and see if that helps in any way. If instead of concentrating on getting him to be more active, you could spend some time getting to know how he feels, maybe that would help us to understand why he is refusing to do anything.

**Sheila**: I suppose it won't hurt to try; anything is better than the open warfare which we seem to have at the moment; he really seems angry sometimes.

**Supervisor**: Perhaps if you simply made it clear that you are picking up hidden anger, it just might help him to open up about it. Let's try it and see.

## Discussion

In this session, the supervisor has attempted to facilitate Sheila's examination of her feelings about Ted, and given her an opportunity to be honest and open about them without fear of censure. She has also helped Sheila to make links with her own feelings and thereby hopefully gone some way towards increasing self-awareness. Additionally, the session has raised many issues in relation to attitudes towards ageing and the elderly which will need further discussion in future sessions, but which have been aired usefully here. Crucially, perhaps, the supervisor has picked up the parallel processes in Sheila's experience, those with her own parents and with the elderly people in her care as a nurse and the way in which this patient Ted seems to break the rules in some way.

Obviously, Sheila cannot be simply left floundering with the problems this patient poses and needs some advice, educational input on how to intervene, how to break the deadlock. The supervisor provides this in the form of suggestions for communication with the patient, pointing Sheila towards an emphasis on getting to know Ted, so as better to understand his feelings about his situation. In this simple supervision session, it is possible to demonstrate how self-awareness, attitudes, knowledge and skills can be addressed in a very meaningful way for the supervisee.

## Supervision session two

**Sheila**: I tried what you suggested. It was so hard at first, he simply wouldn't talk to me at all. When I said I thought that perhaps he was very angry about his situation, he simply became more angry with me. I felt awful. On Tuesday, the chap from the lab came to take some more blood from him. He seems to have had tests every day this week. Ted moaned as usual and said he was sick of having all these tests. A week ago, I suppose I would have become a bit impatient with him, I mean he always seems to be holding everything up. But since trying to talk to him, I sort of felt he had a point really, so I said: 'If you don't want to have the blood taken just now, I will ask the chap to come back some other time'. He seemed genuinely appreciative, and said no, it was O.K., thanks anyway. After that, I went back, and he was much more talkative. Apparently, he was made redundant 5 years ago when his firm closed down. He had a very responsible engineering job, and at 59 couldn't get another one. He seems to have sat around brooding about it, feeling pretty miserable ever since. He is extremely worried about the tests; he really thinks he has got something very serious. I couldn't really reassure him that he hasn't because obviously the consultant isn't sure either. He told he he hasn't slept properly since he came in, which no-one seems to have noticed. He also said he felt I didn't like him; that made me feel dreadful.

**Supervisor:**   Dreadful that he had noticed, or dreadful that you couldn't disguise it better? After all, nurses are not supposed to have negative feelings about patients, are they? How did you react when he said he thought you didn't like him?

**Sheila:**   Well, what could I say? I sort of denied it and said that he mustn't mind me when I am busy.

**Supervisor:**   I wonder if more might have been gained by being a bit more honest about the effect he has on you when he is grumpy and refuses to do things for himself? Sounds as if he has been feeling depressed and sorry for himself for the last five years without having to face the effect that might have on other people. However, it is also important that you recognize the reality of his feelings: for example, his fear of being seriously ill, which seems mixed up in his feelings of uselessness.

   I wonder if anyone has asked him for any help in the past 5 years; I wonder if he has felt needed by anyone. Perhaps you could help by being more honest about how you would like him to help you and himself, instead of simply storing up resentment. This may be a way of getting him to examine how he interacts with his family when he is at home.

**Sheila:**   Since I have tried a bit harder to talk to him, I feel a bit more for him now. It seems to help to get to what is behind his behaviour. I have managed to talk to him about the tests more; he was so hostile before that he wasn't really getting a full explanation of what was going on. I suppose he felt more isolated and frightened because he wasn't really being kept informed.

**Supervisor:**   I suppose also that when we do not know what is going on and we are frightened and worried, it can all seem worse if everything appears to be out of our control. Lots of things in the past 5 years have probably seemed out of Ted's control since the redundancy. I think that the small act of saying he didn't need to have his blood taken if he didn't want to in some small way said to Ted: 'You are still in control'. I suppose a lot of people who are getting older, with failing health, can very easily feel that loss of control. I suppose you are a person who likes most things under control yourself; on the ward, for instance, or with your parents: if they failed to cope with getting older, would it pose a problem for your control?

**Sheila**: I don't really know, but with Ted it was as if nothing we did could help. When patients are very physically ill or dying, you can feel useful, you know what to do for them. I didn't know what to do for Ted; he just seemed angry about getting old. There just doesn't seem to be much point in that.

**Supervisor**: I suppose when we have very positive examples of coping in our own life, like your parents, it is difficult to see that something might prove a very negative experience for other people. We don't help by denying their right to feel that way. I wonder if you have any ideas of going a bit further with Ted before he is discharged.

**Sheila**: Well, obviously, a great deal will depend on the results of the tests, but even so I think he needs to talk a lot more about how he feels. I suppose it's no use us finding him something to do; the important thing is that he should find something he wants to do and be in control of his situation. I have talked to him about not sleeping; he says he doesn't want any more pills, so I have taught him how to use a relaxation tape before he tries to get to sleep. Apparently it's helping, and he even laughed about it the other day. I have managed to get him to talk to another patient in the ward, a fellow engineer, much older than Ted but quite capable of a reasonable conversation. I think that is making him feel useful in some small way. I suppose in the next week I should continue to get to know him, and then try to talk to him about what he thinks things are going to be like when he goes home. Maybe he could see some changes he might like to make, with some help. I wondered after talking to him more if maybe he wasn't a bit depressed. If his mood doesn't change much before he goes home, I may talk to him about having a chat with the liaison psychiatric nurse.

## Discussion

In most cases, patients are only in hospital for a short time, as in Ted's case, and supervision can make all the difference between the nurse becoming trapped in a reaction which is destructive both to the patient and to herself. Supervision can help the nurse not simply to view all the clinical alternatives in the care of individual patients, but also to identify blocking features which are transferred into the nursing situation from her own personal experience.

The simple use of supervision in the case of Ted allowed the nurse to examine her intervention, her professional and personal attitudes to ageing and the elderly, and to become more aware of the influence of deeply held personal ideals and the manner in which she was transferring them on to the patients in her charge. In the longer term, it might also have the effect of stimulating her into a closer examination of some of the issues in her own life, but that is a bonus and not the objective of supervision in nursing.

## CASEWORK CONVERSATION TWO

### Background

Alan is a psychiatric nurse undertaking the ENB course in Community Psychiatric Nursing. He is a young man of 28, married, and has recently had his first child. He and his wife are delighted with their new baby daughter. Alan is on placement as part of the course requirements. He has started to see a lady who is complaining of depression and anxiety in counselling sessions. This woman's brother committed suicide in adolescence some years ago, and only now does this seem like a huge issue for her. She is married with two grown-up daughters, one of whom is about to be married.

Alan has presented his casework material in the form of audio-tapes in group supervision sessions.

### Supervision session

**Patient**:   I feel so anxious, I just can't seem to relate it to anything.

**Alan**:   Have you felt anything in particular since we met with your husband last week?

**Patient**:   I will tell you something: I felt more relieved, now that Peter had learned something about my feelings that he didn't know before. The bad pregnancies I got through him. And the fact that I didn't get any support when my Gran died. I mean, she brought me up. Everything was shut off.

**Alan**:   You say the bad pregnancies you got through him. It sounds as if you are almost blaming him. How does that make you feel towards him? Why do you feel the blame lies with him?

**Patient**: He was never there when I needed him. I feel very bitter, very bitter. When I had the last miscarriage, it was only pure luck that I started with the pain before he went out. He was a great footballer, he was more interested in going out to the football. He was on his way out of the door, it was only when he heard me screaming with pain that he came back, otherwise I would have been in a right mess with two babies as well.

**Alan:** Are you still bitter towards him?

**Patient:** I feel you can't wipe out the past. I have felt suicidal lately. (in tears)

**Alan:** Is that why your brother's suicide is raised so strongly for you at the moment.

**Patient:** Probably. I always felt that him and me were two of a kind, and that we didn't really fit into the family. I feel as though I have been robbed of something. The doctor wants the girls to leave me alone for most of the day in future, but I feel really frightened, I can't explain it, I feel terrified.

**Alan:** What is that fear about?

**Patient:** I don't know. I just feel that I am in fear of losing something and I don't know why. I feel as if I am going to lose Pete (husband) and I don't know why. I have no reason to feel like this.

**Alan:** Is it I wonder because you feel other people have been snatched away from you?

**Patient:** I feel as though everything I have ever truly really loved has been snatched away from me, yes. Even when I lost my Gran, I mean it was normal, she was 86, but I felt robbed. Even when I am with Peter now, I am not sure, not really sure that he loves me. I felt bitter about my Gran going; selfish, really, isn't it?

I always thought I was so sure of myself, always got on with people, I don't know why I should feel like this. It's morbid feelings really, a feeling that something bad is going to happen. Sort of always waiting for something frightening to happen.

**Alan:** It is a fear.

**Patient:** Yes.

**Alan:** And the only sense you seem to make of it is that you are going to lose something else.

**Patient:** Yes. But it's all so stupid really. I have got two lovely girls, one of them is getting married in July; I don't want anything to spoil it, and yet I cannot get into it at all.

**Alan**: Is it perhaps bringing back memories of your own wedding?

**Patient**: Not really. There is nothing to remember, we were in and out of the registry office. I was pregnant, we had to live with my parents for a while. I wasn't allowed to sit in the living room because I was a disgrace. My father said I was like one of those girls in the *News of the World*. My mother never supported me, just like she never supported my brother Jeff. My sister and I used to have to listen to my stepfather arguing and hitting him, and she would never say a word.

**Alan**: How does that make you feel about your mother?

**Patient**: Sad, very sad. Sad that she never listened to us when we tried to tell her.

## Discussion

It is very obvious simply from this initial snatch of dialogue that Alan and the patient had very quickly established rapport and a 'common feeling language'. Consequently, the material being shared by the patient is of a fairly deep emotional nature. In particular, this woman's feelings are in almost total contrast to the situation of domestic bliss and new parenthood which is seemingly the case for Alan and his wife at present.

During supervision, the supervisor first of all asked Alan how he felt he had coped and whether he was concerned about anything in particular in relation to the case. This allowed Alan to discuss his feelings about the session and the case generally in a safe, non-judgemental atmosphere. One of the most important contributions clinical supervision can make to nursing is to allow supervisees to be honest about their feelings of ability to handle a case. This is particularly true when the case contains extremely disturbing emotional material. It is not in the interest of a patient to have a nurse who is out of his/her depth and cannot admit it.

Alan felt the patient was a cause for concern, but he did not feel worried about working with someone expressing suicidal ideas, so long as he had regular supervision. He felt that the patient was depressed but not suicidally so; in his opinion, they were managing to build a rapport, and the patient was willing to work on her feelings.

The supervisor then pointed out to Alan some of the effective links and interventions he had managed to make. It is a vital part of the supervision process to affirm the supervisee in order to produce a safe and trusting environment in which more sensitive issues can be explored.

Eventually, the supervisor asked Alan why he thought it might be difficult for him to stay with this woman's feelings, and pointed to a couple of occasions when he had actually been more willing to talk to her about others, such as her mother or husband, than to allow her to talk about her own feelings. The supervisor particularly focused on the point she made about bad pregnancies, and on Alan sounding a little piqued that she should blame her husband for her experiences.

Alan said that he thought the material about pregnancies was perhaps a bit close to home for him and 'rang a few bells'. Although he and his wife were absolutely delighted with their new daughter, the pregnancy had been somewhat traumatic and the birth a little difficult. Moreover, his wife was expressing less satisfaction just lately with being at home all day and was anxious to get back to work; he felt that he was somehow blamed for this situation. He was also quite keen to have other children and yet felt a little worried about the idea of his wife going through another difficult pregnancy. He thought some obvious parallels could be drawn between his attempts to avoid discussing some of these issues at home, and not feeling comfortable with the patient's feelings in the session.

Alan said that, although he could sympathize with the woman in some ways, it all felt a little bit unreasonable, after all, she did have everything she wanted, and yet was still feeling terrible. He knew this was not a 'professional' attitude, but had to admit to being irritated by the patient occasionally. 'I mean, her daughters are having to look after her; it's a bit much, and the doctor has quite rightly told her it must stop.' The supervisor then asked Alan to think about his own value systems, in particular the ones he would apply to women who are mothers, his wife for example. Alan identified that he did see motherhood as a privilege, and tended to regard it only in a fairly positive light. He even admitted to feeling a little irritated with his wife of late when she complained about being bored at home. When he kissed the baby goodbye every morning, he frequently thought how good it would be to look after her instead of having to go to work.

A discussion ensued on the sociological factors influencing women's experience of motherhood. Alan said that, whilst he had 'done' sociology as part of his training, including the present course, it made more sense when you could actually apply it to an issue which was important in a case.

The remainder of the supervision session was occupied with discussing those loss issues the patient had raised with Alan and what possible meanings and impact they could have for her. Alan was helped to look at these issues as they influenced the patient's life now: feelings of loss of love, having to face the absoluteness of past losses, and the inability to put right what has always been wrong in parental relationships. The supervisor asked Alan if he thought that dealing with a vulnerable, depressed woman who regarded her past experience as a series of unfeeling relationships and losses, held any particular dangers for a male nurse. Alan very quickly identified some worries he had about how the patient was perhaps perceiving him. He had noticed that she frequently used his name in a pleasant, almost flirtatious way. And once or twice, when he had shown what he saw as normal concern for her feelings, she had commented on the difference between Alan and Pete, her husband. Alan felt that she saw him as a sort of 'new man' who understood and empathized with the female condition. Indeed, that was how he liked to see himself. Discussing the issue in supervision, however, had helped him to see that the patient was sometimes putting on a flirtatious tone in order to flatter a desired image he had of himself. One of the ways to handle this would be to talk about these comparisons she overtly made, in an attempt to give her some insight into the idealistic fantasy she held of Alan and the reasons why she felt she was not getting emotional support, especially from Pete. Alan agreed to stay alert to this and to try the suggested intervention at the earliest opportunity.

## CASEWORK CONVERSATION THREE

### Background

Claire is a 30-year-old community nurse, married with no children. Her special responsibility is to provide advice and support to HIV-positive haemophiliacs and their families. She is based on the haematology unit where patients spend a lot of time attending for various treatments; she provides support to patients in the unit as well as visiting them in their homes. Many of the people Claire deals with are very young men, some of them teenagers. A few of her patients are now developing AIDS and dying. This is causing a great deal of distress for everyone concerned in their treatment, and Claire has found herself providing support for the staff as well as the patients and their families.

She is currently deeply involved with the home nursing care of a young man of 17 years, Jeremy, who is now quite ill and not expected to survive much longer. Jeremy is a very bright young man of whom great academic achievements were expected; he had also dealt very positively with his severe haemophilia and become quite an exceptional swimmer. He comes from a very close, loving and reasonably affluent family who are all totally devastated by what is now happening to him. Claire's brief is to assist the district nursing team to provide 24-hour care for Jeremy so that his parents can have him at home to die, which is their wish. In the past two weeks, Claire has been spending more and more time with Jeremy, and frequently is still at his home with the parents in the early hours of the morning, in her own time. She has had one or two rows with the district nursing team about what she sees as a poor standard of care, which she feels is simply not good enough. On the last occasion, she ordered the district nurse out of the house and reported her to her manager for what she felt was a display of inappropriate attitudes to Jeremy. Claire has been asked to account for her actions by her senior nurse, and feels very angry that she should have to do so. She has always used supervision effectively in the past, but interestingly has never discussed Jeremy in supervision. She has, however, raised the reprimand by her senior nurse with her supervisor.

## Supervision session

**Supervisor**:   So you feel your manager was wrong not to support you in front of the district nursing manager. What exactly did you expect her to do?

**Claire**:   I have reported to her often enough how stressful it is to work in HIV nursing. I mean, I know she isn't directly involved with the patients, but you would think she would understand that I cannot just let any nurses near the patients. That district nurse didn't like Jeremy, she hardly talked to him; just came in, did his pressure areas, gave his drugs, washed him, made his bed, and then said she had to dash. Said something about having an old patient to see before lunch. Honestly, if they don't want to work in HIV, why on earth do they get into it in the first place?

**Supervisor**:   Did Jeremy say anything to you? You obviously didn't like the nurse's attitude, but I wonder if Jeremy picked up whatever it is you picked up also?

**Claire**:   Well, even if he did, he wouldn't say anything; he is so sweet, he wouldn't want to cause any trouble. He was exactly the same when he was in the unit, never the slightest trouble. I had to complain a number of times about things not being quite right in his room. He would never have said a word.

**Supervisor**:   And his parents, are they quite happy with his care?

**Claire**:   Well, it's the same old story, isn't it? They think all the district nurses are 'angels' and can do no wrong. Also, if anything was neglected, they are so stunned and shocked by what is happening that they wouldn't really notice, unless it stood out like a sore thumb.

**Supervisor**:   It sounds as if you feel that there is only you to make sure everything is all right. I get the impression that you would find it hard to trust Jeremy's care to anyone else. Is that why you are so tired, spending more evenings and nights there when you have finished at the unit?

**Claire**:   Yes, I suppose so. Oh, I know I am doing too much, but who else is going to be there? His parents cannot cope alone, and the district nurses are simply not good enough. Anyhow, Jeremy has got used to me now, we get along so well. I mean, I have known him years, from him coming into the unit for his factor 8 when he was a little boy.

**Supervisor**:   It must be quite an ordeal for you, too, to watch what is happening to him now.

**Claire**:   Oh, it's absolutely dreadful. You know, he used to swim a lot, really well. And it was obvious he was going to do really wonderfully at school: he got ten top grade G.C.S.E.s last year. And now he weighs so little, about six stones; and he can hardly do anything for himself, he is so weak. And the final insult is that he seems to be developing C.M.V. retinitis, which might make him blind if the treatment is not successful. What's even worse to take, sometimes, is the way in which he stays so cheerful and accepting. If it were me, I would be so bloody angry. I mean, it need not have happened. We should have known about the factor 8 earlier.

**Supervisor**:   You sound really disturbed about this, almost as if you are responsible in some way . . .

**Claire** (in tears):   Not just in some way. I am really responsible: I gave Jeremy the infected factor 8 which gave him HIV. I got on so well with him that each time he came in for his treatment I would be the one who gave it to him. He used to laugh and say I was the best nurse on the unit, that it didn't hurt when I did it. God, if only we could have known!

**Supervisor**:   But you didn't know that the factor 8 was contaminated. You were giving it to save Jeremy's life. You know that without it he would certainly have died from the haemophilia.

**Claire**:   Oh, I know all that. But, with all the others who we know have become infected, most of the nurses on the unit gave them their treatment at some time to another, but with Jeremy, it was just me. Because I was special for him.

**Supervisor**:   I suppose you have to be very special for him now; you feel that you must make sure nothing is wrong with his treatment. You feel you must be there and you cannot let him down in any way. Is that how it seems?

**Claire**: He had such faith in me, you see. He would come in the unit when he was just a little fellow and ask for Claire—'Claire doesn't hurt me'. He was a delightful child as well, so clever; he would bring me drawings he had done at school. It is just so horrendous that he is dying now from something I gave him, something he thought would make everything all right.

**Supervisor**: Do you think Jeremy or his family blame you or the hospital for what is happening?

**Claire**: No, not at all. I almost wish they would. They are extremely sensible people who are angry about what has happened, but not with individuals. Certainly not with me; I am like a member of the family almost.

**Supervisor**: You sound as if you would like them to get angry with you, to punish you in some way.

**Claire**: I have never really thought about it like that, but I do feel I have a responsibility to make sure that his care is perfect.

**Supervisor**: Do you think that taking total responsibility for his 24 hour care is the way to achieve 'perfection'?

**Claire**: No, I suppose it isn't really, but I find it hard to trust the district nurses. It's as if I must be there to make sure nothing goes wrong.

**Supervisor**: I guess you felt that Jeremy trusted you once and you let him down in some way. By being there constantly now, you won't let him down again. Is that how it feels?

**Claire**: Yes, like a terrible responsibility and, if I'm honest, a lot of ownership as well. What it comes down to, I suppose, is that I don't like handing his care over.

**Supervisor**: If these feelings were to go on, I think they might even get in the way of the care Jeremy needs. He is going to need I.V. therapy almost everyday now for the C.M.V., isn't he?

**Claire**: I have been very worried about how things are going really; I think I have made the family very dependent on me, and now I am not sure I can cope with it all alone.

**Supervisor**: But there is no need to, is there? It seems to me that the best way forward is to take an honest look at your past relationship with Jeremy, and to be just as honest about it with him, with his family, but most importantly with your district nursing colleagues who are trying to care for him. They can only do so properly if you give them permission and help.

**Claire**:   I know it has got to happen, but it isn't going to be easy. The whole thing has become so complicated.

**Supervisor**:   It wouldn't be easy to continue along the present road either; it has already put you under a great deal of stress, and caused problems with Jeremy's nursing care. I think you will need a lot of support in the next few months to cope with letting go, not simply of his care, but of him as well.

## Discussion

This supervision session provides a good example of the usefulness of supervision as a means of exploring and resolving a conflict situation which has the potential adversely to affect nursing care. What on the surface seemed like a fairly commonplace issue of professional boundaries and interdisciplinary rivalry, is shown in supervision to be much more complicated indeed. Claire's inability to operate effective professional boundaries, and to cooperate fully with other nurses involved in the care of Jeremy, was not due to a lack of knowledge or awareness, but to the influence of unresolved feelings of guilt and responsibility.

Had this issue been dealt with simply on a managerial basis, it could possibly have ended with the need to discipline Claire for her attitude, which would have been most unhelpful both for her and for Jeremy and his family. Besides, Claire would have been very likely to become ill through unresolved conflict.

Supervision had the effect of allowing Claire to talk about her feelings and to begin the 'letting go' of Jeremy which was so vital if she was not going to be devastated by loss and guilt later. Nursing as a profession inculcates feelings of responsibility into its members as a matter of course. We are constantly expected to feel responsible for what happens to 'our patients'. When such responsibility is compounded by something as dreadful as the HIV virus, it should come as no surprise that feelings become complex and confused. Furthermore, when compared with a disciplinary or managerial approach, supervision has the extra advantage of being educational. Claire learned a great deal from discussing her feelings about Jeremy's case and will have much experience to draw on in transferring skills gained from that to other cases.

It was essential to everyone concerned that Claire should be able to get out of the angry position in which she had become stuck. The strength of her feelings could also have made it very difficult for Jeremy and his family to ask for, or gain access to, other appropriate help, and similarly for his family to undertake any preparatory grief work in anticipation of the terrible loss they faced, at a time when Claire was incapable of getting in touch with her own feelings and was rushing around making everything 'perfect'.

As stated at the beginning of this chapter, extracts of 'casework conversations' have been presented as examples of how effective high quality supervision can be in helping nurses to develop skills, attitudes and knowledge. In the opinion of the authors, the cases presented are representative of problems facing the nursing profession every day, such as death and dying, infectious diseases, getting older, attitudes to women and pregnancy. All the cases contain examples of emotional problems and feelings to be faced in the patient, but more importantly, in ourselves. Issues of loss, in particular, are central to most nursing care. The mere fact of illness itself constitutes a whole catalogue of loss, even for the most average, straightforward patient. In the majority of cases, these losses are thankfully shortlived; however, in some cases, they are much more long term and may ultimately mean loss of life, with all its implications. The examples of supervision 'in action' presented here represent positive and adaptive ways of dealing with those feelings.

# CHAPTER SEVENTEEN

# 'Supervision for life'

## Tony Butterworth and Jean Faugier

With the necessary professional framework in place (UKCC, 1990) it is possible to construct a model which will provide clinical supervision throughout our working lives as nurses. Given that certain preconditions are present and that sufficient time is given to allow supervision to grow, then there is no reason why this important activity could not take stronger root in nursing. This chapter provides a composite view of four elements which are central to the provision of a model of 'supervision for life'. These are some ground rules, potential methods, room for growth and support and a composite model.

### SOME GROUND RULES

Readers will recall that in Chapter 1 some ground rules for supervision were presented and it is useful to reconsider them briefly.

1. Skills should be constantly re-defined and improved throughout professional life.
2. Critical debate about practice activity is a means to professional development.
3. Clinical supervision offers protection to independent and accountable practice.
4. Introduction to a process of clinical supervision should begin in professional training and education, and continue thereafter as an integral part of professional development.
5. Clinical supervision requires time and energy and is not an incidental event.

### POTENTIAL METHODS

Potential methods for supervision and mentorship are based on definitions put forward by Houston (1990) and provide a useful model for presenting the ways in which clinical supervision and mentorship might be a regular activity for nurses.

1. Regular one-to-one sessions (with a supervisor from your own discipline or training establishment).
This is a situation where an experienced person can discuss with and comment upon a nurse's potential and ability to be in tune with patients.
It is a well tried device for some branches in nursing but could be developed in others to be less 'criticism focused' and more constructive and enabling as an experience.

2. Regular one-to-one sessions (with a supervisor from a different discipline).
This method may be necessary because it might be that the only person with whom one can have immediate and regular contact is from another discipline. Alternatively, a situation may arise where this individual is the one which inspires most confidence in the supervisee. There will be some inevitable 'culture clashes' and these must be recognized at the outset and discussed.

3. One-to-one peer supervision.
In sessions of this sort opportunity is given for participants to counsel each other, reflect upon practice, and take turns in being the leader for a session.

4. Group supervision (within own discipline).
There is opportunity for group supervision where nurses meet collectively and discuss their activities. Specific time may need to be identified for these sessions and it is not certain for example whether or not 'report giving' is the right time to do this as there are often other pressing concerns to be dealt with. It might be arranged, however, that at predetermined times one nurse could present a patient and discuss the nursing care they are receiving with a group of other nurses of varying experience and seniority.

5. Peer group supervision.
There is no reason why a peer group cannot be used to give some measure of level of performance. Case conferencing is an example in which a nurse will present a patient or a family and receive comment and feedback from peers on their performance and interventions.

6. Network supervision.
This provides a system of presenting a number of one-to-one and peer supervision sessions for a shared review to a more experienced supervisor/facilitator at a 'collective session'. A system of this sort is an

invaluable support where supervision is still developing as part of practice and the participants need feedback on their sessions.

The reader might be forgiven for assuming that this list provides an encouragement to nurses to spend all their time in thoughtful reflection and consequently do no work at all! This is not a recommendation we wish to make, indeed the hard-pressed nurse will have only limited time for any new activity in their busy working day. It serves to remind us however that there are many ways of thinking about and providing supervision but, if we are serious about engaging in clinical supervision and mentorship, a case must be made with employers and senior staff to devote enough time to it, and make it an established part of nursing work.

## WINNING THE RESOURCE ARGUMENT

In the preceding chapters, it has been argued—we believe convincingly—that clinical supervision is a major, if not *the* major force in improving clinical standards, enhancing the quality of care, and ensuring less strain and burnout in nursing staff by encouraging more self-awareness and self-expression. However, even as we write these words, we can hear many a nurse manager echoing the sentiments of Mandy Rice Davis: 'You would say that, wouldn't you?'. It therefore becomes essential to address the financial and resource issues seriously if clinical supervision is to become an accepted and expected part of nursing.

One fairly effective manner in which to get to the hearts of hard-pressed health service managers is via their budgets. In order to convince them of the value of clinical supervision over and above what they may view as anecdotal evidence, they should first be persuaded to build into any provision of clinical supervision an evaluation element which can monitor such variables as staff sickness and time off, increases in innovative practice and expressed consumer satisfaction. Obviously, if such improvements in practice and absence rates can be made with relatively low extra financial outlay, they are bound to prove attractive in these cost cutting times.

The profession has a responsibility to prove the effectiveness of additional practices which may take time and resources. For too long now we have somewhat baulked at this responsibility. If we are seriously offering clinical supervision as a means of improving practice and education in nursing, then it behoves us to find understandable arguments with which to support our claims. Failure to do so would leave us open to the very pertinent accusations of self-indulgence, or therapy on the firm's time.

## THE 'CATCH 22' OF CLINICAL SUPERVISION AND MENTORSHIP

This section could perhaps also take its title from a Joni Mitchell classic hit of the sixties: 'You don't know what you've got till it's gone'. The singer concerned, whom some of our older readers will remember, was bemoaning the loss of her 'old man'. However, the moral holds true for supervision also. Unless nurse managers have themselves undergone the experience of supervision, they will find it very difficult to appreciate what all the fuss is about. This must be a very good argument for starting any programme of mentorship and supervision at the top as well as providing for students and clinically-based staff. Senior nurses and nurse managers also need mentorship and supervision; they frequently have to shoulder quite onerous responsibilities and workloads, not least the pastoral responsibility they must exercise towards a whole range of staff. Personal issues can prove extremely taxing emotionally and face senior managers with difficult decisions. A network of supervision and mentorship established at a level which in no way compromises authority structures is an essential element in assisting senior nurses to cope more effectively with these issues. More and more frequently, such nurses are arranging supervision and mentorship with senior colleagues in neighbouring health districts. Once established and appreciated by senior staff, such a programme can be a tremendous boost to the establishment of supervision and mentorship at other levels in the nursing hierarchy.

## A MODEL OF GROWTH AND SUPPORT

The reader first met this model in Chapter 3. The model recommends a process which encourages personal and educational growth and support for clinical autonomy. Its key requirements ask certain responses from participants:

1. Generosity of time and spirit;
2. Reward through praise and encouragement;
3. Openness to the limitations and imperfections of both supervisor and supervisee;
4. A willingness to learn (no matter how senior or experienced);
5. Being prepared for thought-provoking material but remembering to offer a well considered response;
6. Supervision and mentorship reminds us of our humanity. When we are touched by the joys and sorrows of others it is necessary to maintain the dignity of others and of ourselves.
7. Clinical supervision and mentorship is uncompromising in its clinical and intellectual rigour;
8. Supervision demands sensitivity and trust.

## A COMPOSITE MODEL OF CLINICAL SUPERVISION AND MENTORSHIP

Adapting the model of continuous development suggested by PREP (1990) a model can be demonstrated which captures the ideas expressed in this book.

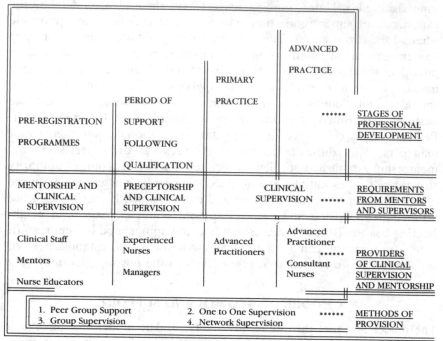

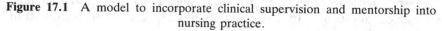

**Figure 17.1** A model to incorporate clinical supervision and mentorship into nursing practice.

## THE MODEL IN ACTION

The following are examples taken from actual experiences of supervision in practice. They show how supervision may be used in a group or as an individual and the impact it can have on nursing care. What these examples also hopefully demonstrate is that the impulse for supervision can be generated equally from the top (managers) or from below (student nurses).

## The student nurse's tale

Alex is a second-year student nurse working on a care of the elderly unit.

He is undertaking general nurse training and on the whole is enjoying it. The unit on which he is placed at the moment is seen as a flagship in care of the elderly within his hospital, and managers and tutorial staff regard it as a really well run and innovative unit providing high standards of care. Alex has already completed eight weeks of a 12-week placement and, whilst there is much to praise and lots to learn, he is troubled by an underlying unhappiness among the clinical ward staff. In staffroom discussions, many of the trained nurses complain about the pace of change on the unit and the increasing demands being made upon them to be more and more innovative in raising standards and thereby the profile of the unit in the hospital. When he sees the nurse manager or his nurse tutors, Alex finds it impossible to voice his concern because they begin their conversations with him by telling him how lucky he is to have a placement on such a forward thinking unit. Alex finds himself caught between a real admiration for the changes and innovations which are being tried, and a feeling that those in charge have an unrealistic view of life on the unit and do not understand the perspectives of the nursing staff. This is an unpleasant situation, and he is unable to talk about the problems without feeling that he is criticizing the 'favourite child' of senior nurses. He has also noticed that, since the speedy implementation of primary nursing, many of the trained staff are showing the strain. For him personally, it has meant a reduction in opportunities to talk through his placement because they are so very busy. A major disappointment for him has been the realization that many of the trained staff are becoming less and less committed to the changes, frequently describing them as 'theirs', which implies ownership of the innovations by the senior nurses.

It seems to Alex that the person who bridges the management/clinical divide is Susan, the clinical nurse specialist to the unit. Alex discusses his feelings with her and she listens without the need to be defensive in any way. Susan also says that she is very impressed by the time Alex has taken analysing the malaise developing on the unit, and that she herself had felt that some of the old enthusiasm was declining of late (reward through praise, and demonstrating a willingness to learn). Susan suggests that regular supervision groups might at least enable the nurses on the unit to talk openly about their fears in relation to innovation and change. After discussing the idea with everyone involved, it was agreed to enlist the support of a senior colleague from psychiatry experienced in supervision groups and senior enough to feel comfortable challenging senior nursing colleagues if necessary.

*Generosity of time and spirit.* To establish the group as a working supervision vehicle, everyone had to be committed enough to give up time. Nursing management in particular had to see the group as important enough to set time aside for it and ensure their own attendance. Only by adopting the right spirit and putting to one side feelings of threat or doubts about motives could the group succeed. This requires a generosity of spirit on all sides, an approach to the group which is positive.

*Reward through praise and encouragement.* It is essential that the supervisor, in this case the nurse running the group, recognizes the risks involved for people entering supervision and sets the agenda by openly acknowledging the difficulties we all have in giving up our well developed defences.

The coming together of clinical and senior nurses in a supervision group for the ultimate benefit of improved relationships hopefully leading to improved patient care is a very adult, professional act, and should be rewarded as such.

*Openness to the limitations and imperfections of both supervisor and supervisee.* One of the most important lessons of clinical supervision, whether conducted in a group or individually, is the quickly dawning realization that the supervisor does not have all the answers.

Difficulties can also arise when the development of more self-awareness leads us to realize how much influence our own personal agendas have on our professional responses. In the case of the unit being described here, a senior charge nurse had ultimately to accept that he was failing to give the changes in the unit as much support as they deserved primarily because he had been unsuccessful in obtaining a promotion recently. This coming to terms with our personal imperfections can be a slow and difficult business.

*A willingness to learn.* During the course of the first few meetings, it was obvious that there was some anger in particular towards the unit manager Peter, who was seen as the major driving force behind the many good ideas which were being presently implemented on the unit. This nurse is a graduate with experience in clinical nursing research. The group faced him with the difficult lesson that simply having the ideas and believing you are right is not sufficient to maintain the commitment of other nursing staff and the smooth running of the unit. He was given the chance, via the medium of supervision, to examine in a positive atmosphere the mistakes he had made in attempting to impose change without consideration for other members of staff, surely a far better way of resolving the issues than the brewing confrontation imminent when Alex was first placed on the unit.

*Being prepared for thought-provoking material.* During the supervision sessions, it became apparent to the senior staff and especially Peter, the unit manager, that many of the sentiments being expressed by the clinical staff centred on his recent promotion, with the idea that many of the changes in patient care and innovative practices on the unit were nothing more than other items for his and others' C.V.s. This caused some distress and challenged the impression that he had of himself as a selfless professional. With the help of the supervisor, he was able rationally to consider some of this material and recognize that, due to a basic lack of involvement from others, many of the changes could quite easily be viewed in that manner, even though consciously he was convinced he had acted solely in the interests of better patient care. Reflection and consideration by the group also led everyone to conclude that there is nothing wrong in furthering one's career through pursuing excellence in patient care. When looked at like this, much of the resentment about Peter's promotion was effectively dealt with.

*Supervision and mentorship reminds us of our humanity.* During one of the early supervision sessions, the supervisor commented that Elaine, one of the enrolled nurses, always intervened in order to suggest a return to the old ways of doing things. The supervisor asked if Elaine was unhappy on the unit. Elaine responded very tearfully saying that the last 12 months had been absolutely awful, that everything had changed so fast she did not feel that she was keeping up. Most of the charge nurses and sisters had only qualified relatively recently and all seemed able to cope with the demands of primary nursing. She felt that it was an admission of failure to tell anyone and had therefore kept it all to herself. The group was very supportive and all felt that they should have had some way of recognizing before a year had gone by that a colleague was struggling with change and was very unhappy. Supervision provided the opportunity for Elaine to show her vulnerability and for others to respond with humanity and care because they recognized their own also.

*Clinical supervision is uncompromising in its clinical and intellectual rigour.* The supervisor listened to all the manifest reasons for the resistance to change being expressed by the group. However, the latent content of their communication seemed to suggest that changes involving primary nursing and greater involvement with the patient as an individual are simply more difficult emotionally and the group had been given little support for this. When Judy, the staff nurse, said how hard it was finding the time and the staff to do things the way the managers recommended, the supervisor suggested that she might find it difficult to be with the patients when they are very ill and when they are dying. At this, Judy became very distressed and said that sometimes, when a patient died, she could not help crying and the distress of the relatives and loved ones stayed with her for hours, even when she went home. Others then felt able to say how hard it was sometimes when you have become very close to a patient. The supervisor was later able to facilitate a discussion which allowed the group to recognize that what they needed was support and supervision rather than distance from the patients.

*Supervision demands sensitivity and trust.* During the group meetings, the nurses involved disclosed feelings about themselves and others, as well as their personal and professional life. Such sharing and disclosure is essential if individuals and teams are to grow emotionally and professionally. In order for such openness to flourish, however, the supervisor must create an atmosphere of trust and sensitivity by the way in which she/he treats the material offered by the group. In this case, the supervisor also helped this process by spending much of the first session laying ground rules of confidentiality with the group.

## The manager's tale

Dennis had only been in post as unit general manager for the Community Nursing Services in his area for six months and he knew he was already feeling the strain. He seemed to be rushing to meet one deadline after another, he was taking more and more work home with him and he did not seem to have any time at all to reflect on what he was actually doing.

He recalled a time when he had worked as a CPN years before and things had reached the same pitch. Then, his manager had provided him with clinical supervision. In that particular district, there had been a strong tradition of clinical supervision within the psychiatric services and everyone received some form of supervision or support. Dennis remembered how useful the time spent in supervision had been, giving him time and space to reflect on priorities and any particularly worrying clients he might have. He did not see why supervision should be reserved for those involved in clinical work alone, and resolved to suggest supervision for managers at his next management meeting. At the back of his mind was a slight concern that he may be the only one feeling the strain and that the other managers might see him as unfit for the job. However, he felt so bad that he was beyond caring and was not prepared to let some misguided sense of pride or embarrassment get in his way.

Dennis quickly found that he need not have worried: his courage in raising the issue of support and supervision for managers gave all his colleagues the opening they had needed to voice concerns about how they themselves were coping.

The personnel manager was given the task of liaising with a neighbouring authority and working out an exchange of expertise in order to provide adequate support and supervision. Their own experience of having a little time in which to review performance and to place issues in perspective meant that the matter of supervision for all grades of clinical staff was quickly on the agenda with widespread support from the nursing management.

Such an initiative not only enhanced the efficiency of nursing management by having the effect of reducing stress, it also provided them with a rare insight into the needs for supervision and support of those working in the clinical area.

There is nothing to prevent any of the ideas shown here from being drawn into nursing in its various specialist manifestations; indeed, many of them are to be found there already. Not to capitalize on such beginnings would be a great waste of potential:

When it seems that a new man or a new school has invented a new thing, it will only be found that the gifted among them have secured a firmer hold than usual of a known thing. (Sickert)

## REFERENCES

Houston, G. (1990) *Supervision and Counselling*, The Rochester Foundation, London.
United Kingdom Central Council for Nursing, Midwifery and Health Visiting (1990) *The Report of the Post-Registration Education and Practice Project*, UKCC, London.

# Index